Food Truck Cookbook

Street Food Recipes

Author

Carla R. Burton

Contents

INTRODUCTION

If there's a better way to spend a summer than on a meandering road trip, I really can't imagine what it would be. Iced tea in the cup holder. Air conditioner working overtime. Stopping for a farm stand peach or a great photo on a whim. And when that road trip just happens to wind its way through the South, with stops along the way for street food from some of America's most imaginative chefs and culinary artists . . . well, that's the sort of summer that's pretty tough to top.

This book is the result of that summer—weeks spent on the road, stopping at festivals, outdoor concerts, beaches, town squares, city street corners, the parking lots of office parks, and pretty much any other place where a tiny kitchen on wheels could find a place to park for long enough to dish up a chalkboard menu's worth of foods that can be enjoyed from a paper tray. Pssst . . . here's a secret: there aren't many foods that *can't* be enjoyed that way.

The best part of my journey? That's easy. It's the abundance of recipes these food truckers shared for this collection.

When I started this project, I was surprised by two of the responses I sometimes heard from friends and family: "There are food trucks in the South? Really? That's cool. Enough for a whole book? Wow"; and "What's a food truck? You mean like a delivery truck?"

I got pretty good at answering these questions.

First of all, yes. Yes, there *are* food trucks in the South. Hundreds of them! Second, if you're reading this right now, I feel pretty confident you know what a food truck is . . . but just in case, a food truck is a large delivery- or RV-style vehicle with a kitchen built right into it and a window for customer ordering and serving.

Previously, only certain parts of this country really knew the delight of street dining. Californians have been buying tacos out of Airstream trailers for decades, and New Yorkers have been noshing on hot dogs from stainless steel carts for even longer. But during the last decade (oh, hallelujah!), the notion of street food has crept inward from the coasts, giving the rest of us a taste of this culinary tradition.

The great thing about Southern food trucks is that they're often run by people who've lived and worked in places outside the South. There's the truck in Atlanta run by a couple who love sharing the flavors they embraced while living in Central America. Now they're fusing Latin flavors with fried green tomatoes, watermelon, and pork ribs.

There's the guy in Little Rock who'd worked in restaurants and country clubs for years, but discovered what he truly enjoyed was making Chinese-style pork buns for his friends, who inspired him to bring those buns to the masses.

Food trucks are cropping up all over the place. From Charleston to Memphis, Louisville to Birmingham, entrepreneurial cooks are dishing up familiar flavors and experimenting with new ideas in their tiny mobile kitchens.

Many of these food truckers have held jobs far beyond anything even remotely related to food service; but they've seen the street food tradition take root in other places, and they've been brave enough to ask, "Why not in the South too?" I met a former carpet salesman, commercial real estate broker, animal rescue worker, medical coder, teacher, and paramedic. They're all food truckers now.

And, of course, there are plenty of industry iconoclasts—those restaurant chefs and culinary school grads who just wanted to break out of the windowless restaurant kitchens and interact with their customers. I heard it dozens of times: "There's nothing better than getting to watch your customers take that first bite."

Roughly estimated, there are at least five hundred food trucks/carts throughout the Southeast region, including Arkansas, Alabama, Tennessee, Georgia, South Carolina, Louisiana, Mississippi, North Carolina, Virginia, West Virginia, and Kentucky. Whether they're serving up comfort food classics or ethnic-inspired specialties, these mobile restaurants are providing another way for the South to enjoy local culinary talent.

I should probably stop here and provide a bit of a disclaimer. You may get to the end of this book and find yourself wondering why your favorite food truck isn't included. There are, after all, some very strong feelings around which truck is THE BEST in every city. It is possible that your favorite truck politely declined to be included, or maybe I wasn't able to catch up with them. Food truckers are busy folks! Please know that any glaring omissions aren't intentional. While the food trucks in this book are particular favorites of mine, I urge you to explore every food truck in your community—not just the ones I've profiled.

I am not a former chef or high-profile culinary expert. I'm just an eater—a massively experienced one. Studying recipes has always enhanced the eating experience for me. I've long loved the quiet luxury of stealing away with a cookbook and discovering how flavors can reach their full potential. Of course, getting in the kitchen is the most important part of that discovery, and I hope these recipes will push you to do just that in your own kitchen. These recipes are crowd-pleasers, by the way. They're the sorts of dishes you'll become known for among your family and friends. Your personal masterpiece could very well be right here in this book!

Most important, though, I hope *The Southern Food Truck Cookbook* helps to spread the food truck gospel in the South. If you're not already eating at the food trucks in your community, it's time to get out there. The menus on these trucks are a gorgeously delicious homage to the foods we've always loved here, and the foods we've yet to discover. So, hit the street, and get to eatin', y'all! When you're done there, head home and see what you can create in your own kitchen!

AN EATER'S GUIDE TO SOUTHERN FOOD TRUCKS

Mobile dining is not restaurant dining. And that is a-ok. While food trucks each have different approaches to service, street noshing is a unique experience altogether. Here are some tips to help you enjoy it.

RECONSIDER "SOUTHERN." So, yes. This is *The Southern Food Truck Cookbook*, but you better think again if you're imagining two thousand miles of nothing but fried chicken and barbecue. Yes, you'll discover remarkable renditions of regional mainstays, alongside new interpretations of old favorites *and* cuisine that has absolutely nothing to do with downhome comfort food. In a region that is rapidly upping its culinary game, this is great news for our dear sweet South. The definition of Southern food is constantly changing these days. Get excited!

PUSH YOUR PALATE. While most food trucks can certainly accommodate culinary scaredy cats, force yourself to be brave. Sure, you could order the base-model grilled cheese, and it'll probably be terrific; but don't cheat yourself out of a more memorable experience. Food truckers are food truckers for a reason—they're inventive types whose best work is usually well beyond the norm. Savor their creativity.

BE SOCIAL. The single best way to establish a bond with food trucks in any area is via Facebook and Twitter. This is where the majority of truckers post their locations, daily specials, and upcoming event appearances. Using social media to follow the food truck scene in your community really pays off when you find yourself craving that brown butter and sage gnocchi you had at the truck down the street last month. Tweet that trucker, and plead for a gnocchi encore. A bonus: Food truckers are often devilishly clever on Facebook and Twitter. Prepare to be charmed!

WATCH YOUR WATCH. Just because a food truck serves lunch from 11 to 3 doesn't mean you can mosey up to the window at 2:30 and still have your pick of the menu. Food trucks almost always have limited quantities of everything—particularly those daily specials. Arriving as close to opening as possible is just plain smart. It's crushing to order that double-decker chocolate gravy biscuit extravaganza listed on the menu board, only to discover that the lucky dog in line ahead of you got the last one.

BRING CASH, BUT DON'T BE SURPRISED IF YOU DON'T NEED IT. The majority of trucks can accept your favorite credit card via those nifty smartphone processing systems. Three cheers for those guys! Still, a few cash-only trucks remain, bless their hearts; so make like a Boy Scout and be prepared. Regardless of how you fork over the money, I think you'll find food truck prices to be a pleasant little bargain for the caliber of food you'll receive in exchange.

SHOUT, SHOUT, LET IT ALL OUT. Food truck kitchens usually run on a generator. Generators can be fairly loud, as can the clanging and commotion of the food prep area. Depending on the noise level in and around a food truck, don't be surprised if you have to shout your order to the guy or gal at the window. It's all part of the mobile dining experience.

SPREAD THE LOVE. Where there is one food truck, there are usually several others. Try them all—in one meal! Grab a hibiscus iced tea at one truck to get started, order pork empanadas at another truck, and round it out with a big salad full of juicy Southern produce (peaches! tomatoes! corn!). Food truckers, especially in the summer, can work some serious magic in the salad department. Eat it up!

EMBRACE THE CONCRETE. Here's a fact: dining at a food truck often means you're responsible for finding your own seating. If you're really lucky, maybe you'll find yourself in a city with a fancy food truck park (Hello, Atlanta!) or a farmers' market (Hello, Nashville!), complete with picnic tables and big umbrellas. Other times you'll fall so madly in love with a truck's spicy shrimp ceviche that you won't even mind chowing down on a park bench or in the front seat of your car. Trust me on this one.

ADMIRE THE TRUCKERS. It may sound hokey, but food truckers—9 times out of 10—are dreamers who weren't afraid to try something different. Some of them left six-figure salary jobs. Others spent years working for other people in restaurant kitchens. Some just wanted a complete career change. The sentimentalist in me really likes helping a dreamer succeed. So if you don't have the guts to quit that job you don't love, let yourself live vicariously through these food truckers!

RECIPES

ELOTES

(MEXICAN CORN ON THE COB)

Makes 8 servings.

Gather it up

8 ears of corn, husks and silks removed

Wooden sticks

1 cup mayonnaise*

1 cup crumbled queso fresco cheese

4 tablespoons chili powder**

Lime wedges, for serving

Make it happen

Bring a large pot of water to a boil and add the ears of corn. Boil for 8 minutes. Remove each ear from the water, and holding the corn with a clean towel, stab the wooden stick into the flat end of the corn. Spread the corn liberally with mayonnaise and dust each ear with the crumbled queso fresco and chili powder to taste. Serve with lime wedges.

* Max prefers to make his own mayonnaise and grind his own peppers for this recipe, but prepared ingredients in this recipe will still yield a delicious result.

** Preferably fresh ground from your favorite chile—dried Pulla or New Mexico peppers work well because of their light heat.

PORK BELLY CARNITAS

Makes 4 to 6 servings.

Gather it up

1 pound pork belly, ideally with the rind on

1 medium onion

4 dried guajillo chiles*

1 tablespoon whole black peppercorns

1 tablespoon whole cumin

2 teaspoons whole coriander

1 bay leaf

Salt

Vegetable oil for frying

6 (6-inch) corn tortillas, warmed

Make it happen

Preheat the oven to 350 degrees.

Cut the pork belly into 1-inch pieces and place in a heavy pot with a lid. Roughly chop the onion and add to the pot along with the chile peppers, black peppercorns, cumin, coriander, bay leaf, and salt. Add enough water to just almost cover the pork. Bring to a simmer on the stove over medium-low heat and cover with the lid. Place in the oven. Braise the pork until it's meltingly tender, about 2 to 2 ½ hours. Remove from the oven and pull the pork belly pieces from the liquid. Discard the liquid and refrigerate the pork until cool. Pour ½ inch oil in a skillet and heat over medium-high to 300 degrees. Shallow-fry the pork and cook on both sides until crispy. Remove the pork from the skillet and add to the warmed tortillas.

* You can find these dried chiles in most grocery stores now, but feel free to substitute ancho chiles if you can't find them.

Max says: "At Holy Molé, we 'smear' the fried pork onto our tortillas in order to spread it out over the tacos."

FRIED FISH

Makes 4 servings.

Gather it up

Vegetable oil for frying

1 tablespoon cumin

2 teaspoons coriander

1 cup masa harina*

1 tablespoon salt

2 tablespoons chili powder, preferably fresh ground

1 pound fish (catfish, cod, tilapia, or haddock), cut into 1-inch pieces

Make it happen

Preheat a deep fryer or a large, deep-sided cast-iron pan to 375 degrees. If using the pan, pour enough oil to deep-fry the fish. In a dry skillet over medium-high heat, toast the cumin and coriander until fragrant and browned slightly. Grind the cumin and coriander. Combine the cumin, coriander, masa harina, salt, and chili powder in a medium bowl. Dredge the fish in the masa harina mixture and fry for about 1 ½ minutes until golden brown and cooked through.

Masa harina is available in the Mexican food aisle at most grocery stores.

PICKLED RED ONIONS

Makes 3 cups.

Gather it up

2 cups red wine vinegar

2 tablespoons sugar

2 tablespoons salt

2 teaspoons oregano

2 teaspoons whole cumin seeds

1 or 2 dried chile de arbol*

1 large red onion

Make it happen

In a medium bowl combine the red wine vinegar, sugar, and salt with a whisk until the sugar and salt are dissolved. Add the oregano, cumin, and chile de arbol. Slice the red onion as thinly as possible and add to the vinegar mixture. Let this mixture soak in the fridge for at least 4 hours; overnight is best.

Dried chile de arbol is available in the Mexican food aisle of most grocery stores.

TOMATILLO SALSA

Makes 3 ½ cups.

Gather it up

1 medium white onion

1 pound tomatillos

4 garlic cloves

1 jalapeño pepper

5 New Mexico chiles, optional

Salt to taste

1 bunch cilantro

Make it happen

Preheat the oven for broiling on high heat. Roughly cut the onions and husk the tomatillos. Place the onions, tomatillos, garlic, and jalapeño on a sheet pan and put under the broiler. Broil until everything is charred deeply and the tomatillos have begun to burst. Add the onions and tomatillos to a blender (or molcajete* if you want to keep things really authentic) and blend well. Add water if the mixture is too thick. Add the chiles if desired at this point and transform it to a beautiful, spicy red salsa. Salt to taste and add the cilantro. Pulse in the blender until it is just chopped, *not pureed.*

* A molcajete is a Mexican mortar and pestle made of volcanic stone.

JICAMA SLAW

Makes 8 servings.

Gather it up

1 large jicama, peeled

½ head green cabbage

1 carrot, peeled

1 jalapeño pepper

½ cup Chipotle Aioli (recipe follows)

Make it happen

Thinly slice and julienne the jicama, cabbage, carrot, and jalapeño. Add the Chipotle Aioli and refrigerate at least 1 hour.

CHIPOTLE AIOLI

Makes 1 ½ cups.

Gather it up

1 egg

3 garlic cloves

1 tablespoon white vinegar

3 morita peppers

1 cup vegetable oil

Salt to taste

Make it happen

Add the egg, garlic, vinegar, and moritas to the bowl of a food processor, and process until the peppers are ground. Create an emulsion by slowly adding the oil in a thin stream while the processor is running. Season with salt and thin with water if needed.

AVOCADO SALSA

Makes 2 ½ cups.

Gather it up

1 small white onion

3 garlic cloves

4 ripe avocados

3 ripe tomatillos, husked

1 jalapeño pepper

1 bunch cilantro

Salt to taste

Make it happen

Preheat skillet over medium-high heat. Quarter the onion and place in the dry skillet. Add the garlic and cook until charred. Slice the avocados in half and remove the pit. Scoop out the pulp into the blender. Halve the tomatillos and add to the blender, along with the charred onions and garlic. Halve the jalapeño and remove the seeds if you prefer a milder salsa. Add to the blender and process until smooth. Add the cilantro and pulse to chop the cilantro. Season with salt to taste.

LIL CHEEZERS

LOUISVILLE

Concept: Grilled cheese sandwiches reimagined

lilcheezers.com

 Twitter: @LilCheezers

In every city I visited, it quickly became apparent that the energy of an area's food truck scene could be attributed to a ringleader of sorts, someone who really got the party started. In Lousiville, that person is Matt Davis. It's only been a few years since Matt was a paramedic pondering a career change. He often found himself watching the Food Network, wondering why those zany-looking mobile diners hadn't cropped up anywhere in Louisville yet. In a progressive, walkable, pedestrian-friendly city, food trucks just made sense to Matt.

What should I order?

The Caprese—mozzarella, fresh basil, tomatoes, balsamic reduction, salt, pepper, and garlic on wheatberry bread.

Turns out, the city's antiquated street vending ordinances didn't allow them. So he took up the cause of changing the city's stance on food trucks. Matt testified in Louisville Metro Council meetings, and he established an ongoing dialogue with the city's decidedly pro-food truck leader, Mayor Greg Fischer. And in addition to starting his own truck—the grilled cheese wonder that is Lil Cheezers—Matt cultivated a community for food trucks in Louisville. In addition to kicking his way through the red tape, he organized a website and social media effort, promoting the community of street food in Louisville.

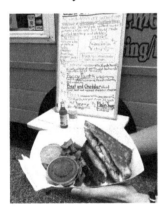

Here's a version of one of Lil Cheezers' most frequently ordered grilled cheese sandwiches. The Fancy Pants is sweet, salty, crunchy, and gooey all at once. Try it for yourself!

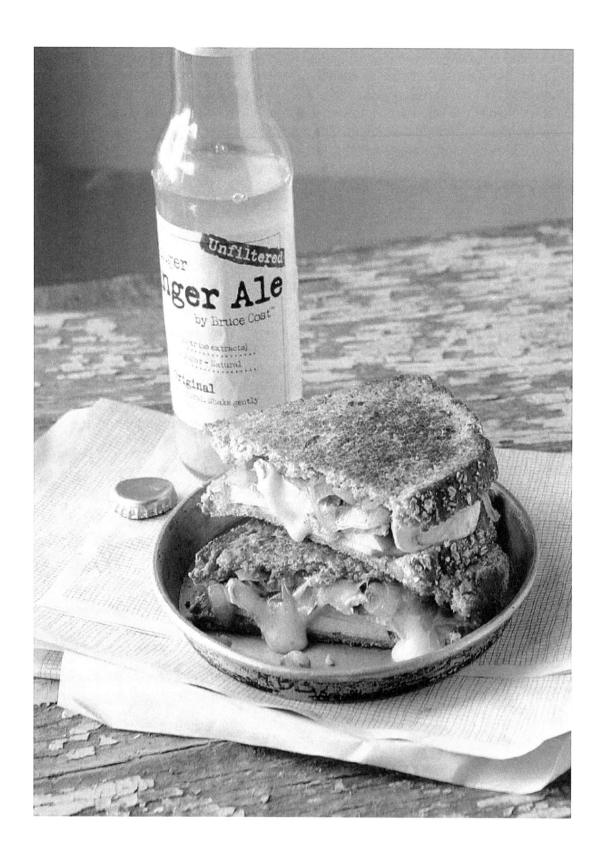

THE FANCY PANTS

Makes 2 sandwiches.

Gather it up

½ tablespoon oil

½ large yellow onion, sliced

Salt to taste

¼ cup butter

4 slices wheatberry bread (the real secret)

⅓ cup chopped walnuts

6 ounces brie, sliced 4 inches long and about ¼ inch thick (six slices total)

1 small Granny Smith apple, thinly sliced

Make it happen

Heat the oil in a skillet over medium heat. Add the onions and salt. Cook until brown, 8 to 10 minutes. Remove from the heat and set aside. Butter each slice of bread and place butter side down on a large skillet or griddle. Arrange the onions on two slices of bread and top each with the walnuts, brie, and apples. Place the remaining two slices of bread on the toppings, and grill each sandwich over medium heat until the bread is golden brown and the brie is melted and gooey.

FRENCH INDO-CANADA

LOUISVILLE

Concept: Poutine and banh mi

 facebook.com/FrenchindoCanada

 Twitter: @IndoCanadatruck

When someone refers to the "holy trinity" in a culinary context, do you immediately think of onions, celery, and bell pepper? Rob Ross doesn't. He thinks of poutine, that magical Canadian mess of French fries ladled with gravy and cheese curds. So he decided to sell it, alongside Vietnamese banh mi sandwiches, out of an old delivery truck that now bears the French Indo-Canada logo.

What should I order?

Why, the poutine, of course! it's the dish Rob Ross claims "changed his life" while visiting our neighbors to the north.

Naturally, the truck's pithy name drew me in, and the concept is, frankly, a bit of a (brilliant) head-scratcher: serving sandwiches from Vietnam along with gravy-smothered fries native to Quebec was too unusual to omit from a book of the Southeast's most memorable food trucks. As Rob describes it, French Indo-Canada is "two former French colonies' take on their former, empirical overlord's cuisine."

It's a delicious, if amusing idea; and not to be hyperbolic, but this collision of cuisines, poutine and banh mi, quite possibly does not exist on any menu anywhere else on earth.

Rob's recipe contribution here is neither for banh mi nor poutine. He opted to send me a chili recipe, which struck me as an unusual choice . . . until I tried the recipe for myself. I can finally stop searching for that elusive 5-star chili recipe. Rob had it all along. You'll notice pretty quickly that this recipe yields far more chili than what you might need for your spouse and 2.5 kids. So invite everyone you know over to your place and serve it up. This could become your own secret recipe! Rob may have shared it, but you don't have to be so generous.

ROB'S THREE-MEAT CHILI

Makes 24 servings.

Gather it up

3 pounds ground turkey

1 pound ground pork

1 pound ground beef

2 poblano peppers, diced

3 jalapeño peppers, finely diced

3 red onions, diced

7 garlic cloves, minced

6 pounds tomatoes, diced (or 6 (15 ounce) cans diced tomatoes)

4 (15-ounce) cans kidney beans, drained

1 (29-ounce) can black beans, drained

⅓ cup toasted cumin seeds

¼ to ⅓ cup granulated garlic

⅛ cup turmeric

¼ cup chili powder (or more depending on your heat preference)

¼ cup paprika

Dried oregano (4 or 5 good shakes)

¼ cup grated 60% dark chocolate

Splash of vinegar

1 can of your finest cheap domestic beer

Kosher salt to taste

Shredded sharp Cheddar cheese, for serving

Saltine crackers, for serving

Make it happen

Rob says: "Get a *giant* stockpot or whatever can hold this much chili."

Heat a large stockpot over medium-high heat. Add the turkey, pork, and beef, and brown. Add the poblano and jalapeño peppers to the pot, cook for a few minutes, and add the onions. When the meat is mostly done, add the garlic cloves.

Allow it to cook until it starts smelling awesome (about 20 minutes) and then add in the tomatoes. Give it a few stirs and toss in the beans. Grind the cumin seeds and add to the pot. Throw in the granulated garlic, turmeric, chili powder, paprika, oregano, chocolate, vinegar, and beer.

Bring it up to a boil, put a lid on it, and turn down the heat to low/medium-low, stirring occasionally. Let it simmer for as long as you can wait, but at least 45 minutes. Salt to taste and serve with shredded sharp Cheddar and saltines.

LOUISVILLE DESSERT TRUCK

LOUISVILLE

Concept: Desserts—any and all! Pies, cakes, cookies, ice cream, etc.

louisvilledesserttruck.com

 Twitter: @LouDessertTruck

I don't know about you, but when I'm chowing down on cake at a wedding reception, I don't really think too much about the person who created it. Pretty thoughtless, huh? But the next time I'm celebrating a lovely couple's nuptials, Leah Stewart will probably cross my mind. That's because for a decade she was never really able to enjoy a summer Saturday away from the wedding cake grind. As one of Louisville's favorite designers of matrimonial confection, Leah often found herself awake for forty-eight-hour stretches, finishing the cakes for multiple weddings in a given weekend.

What should I order?

Turtle sticks! Oh, that sweet and salty duo—pretzel rods dipped in caramel, dipped in chocolate, and rolled in pecans.

A couple years ago Leah decided to take back her Saturdays and channel her baking chops in a different direction. After noticing food trucks popping up throughout the city, she figured it was the perfect time to hit the streets with her own (non-wedding cake) creations.

"It appealed to me on a visceral level," Leah told me during our visit. "I knew I wanted to offer desserts and sweet things, and selling them out of a truck just seemed to fit."

The hometown crowd agrees. When the Louisville Dessert Truck rolls up at a concert, a festival, or outside of Metro Hall, Leah's got a crop of loyals eager to scoop up the treats from her ever-changing menu. Some days she's a cupcakery on wheels. Other days she's a pie wagon. And she's most always an ice-cream truck.

Lucky for you, Leah ponied up her most popular cupcake recipe. I think those newly discovered Saturdays off have put her in a generous mood.

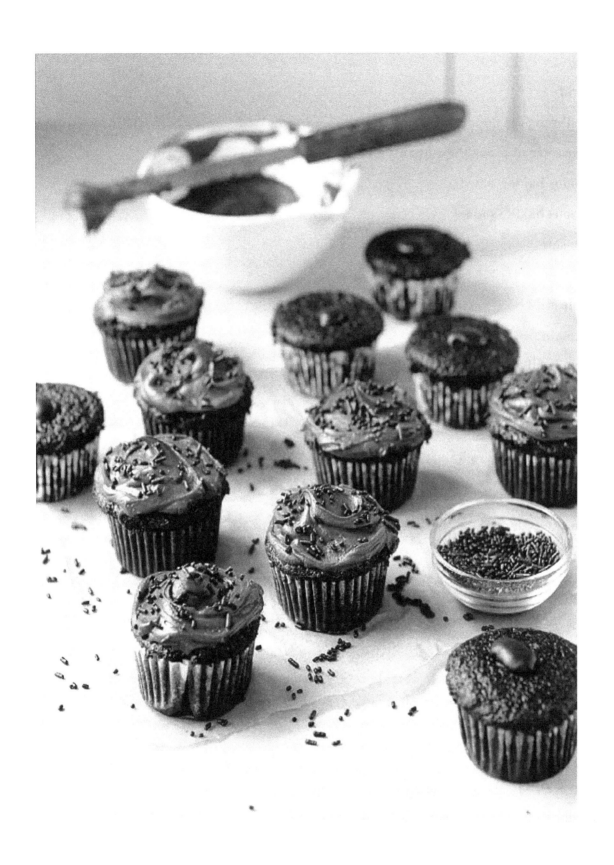

CHOCOLATE × 4 CUPCAKES

Makes 24–27 standard-size cupcakes.

Gather it up

2 cups sugar

1 ¾ cups all-purpose flour

¾ cup unsweetened cocoa (best quality available)

1 ½ teaspoons baking powder

1 ½ teaspoons baking soda

1 teaspoon salt

2 eggs

1 cup whole milk

½ cup vegetable oil

2 teaspoons vanilla extract (best quality available)

1 cup boiling water

Ganache (recipe follows)

Chocolate Icing (recipe follows)

Chocolate sprinkles

Make it happen

Preheat oven to 350 degrees. Line 2 (12-cup) muffin tins with paper liners.

In a large bowl stir together the sugar, flour, cocoa, baking powder, baking soda, and salt. Add the eggs, milk, oil, and vanilla. Beat on medium speed for one minute. Stir in the boiling water. (The batter will be thin, but don't worry. That's how it's supposed to be.) Fill the liners ⅔ full with batter.

Leah says: "I usually put the batter into a large measuring cup with a pour spout and then pour the batter into the liners."

Bake the cupcakes for 18 to 22 minutes. Cool completely on a wire rack.

Put ganache into a piping bag with a large open star tip, plunge it into the top of the cupcake, and squeeze out the ganache as you pull up and away from the cupcake.

Ice the cooled and ganache-filled cupcakes with chocolate icing. Sprinkle chocolate sprinkles on top. The sprinkles are important—they're the fourth layer of chocolate!

Leah says: "You'll ruin a couple until you get the hang of it, but keep trying!"

GANACHE

Makes 2 cups

Gather it up

1 cup heavy cream

9 ounces good-quality semisweet chocolate

Make it happen

Heat the cream to a simmer over medium-high heat. Meanwhile, place the chocolate in a heat-proof bowl. Pour the heated cream over the chocolate, and stir until the chocolate is melted and everything is combined. Allow to cool.

CHOCOLATE ICING

Makes about 2 cups.

Gather it up

½ cup butter or margarine

⅔ cup cocoa powder

3 cups powdered sugar

⅓ cup milk

1 teaspoon vanilla extract

Make it happen

Melt the butter. Stir in cocoa. Alternately add powdered sugar and milk, beating to a spreading consistency. Add a small amount of additional milk, if needed. Stir in the vanilla.

GET IT ON A BUN AT BOOTY'S

LOUISVILLE

Concept: Indulgent comfort food

◪ facebook.com/BootysDiner

Twitter: @BOOTYS2

Get It on a Bun at Booty's is worth a visit, if for no other reason than to meet its proprietress, Tammy Boutiette (pronounced Booty-ay). But there are *plenty* of other reasons to dine at Booty's—the hand-patted burgers, the jerk chicken, the redneck nachos smothered in pulled pork. Tammy (a.k.a. Mrs. Booty) reminds me of that aunt we all have—the one who's always laughing about something, the one who can make a meal that really hits the spot, the one who always has an animated story to tell. As far as stories go, Tammy's got a pretty great one.

What should I order?

Gotta go with the signature Booty Dog! You'll get a smoked sausage smothered in grilled peppers and onions, chili, and Cheddar and Colby Jack cheeses.

Sixteen years ago her husband, Craig (a.k.a. Mr. Booty), came home from work one day and announced they were both quitting their jobs—his as a carpet salesman and hers as a medical coder. The plan? They were going to buy some street food vending carts (think those stainless steel, umbrella-ed hot dog pushcarts) and strike out on their own. The funding? Craig sold his hot tub and Tammy sold her tanning bed. Today their venture has evolved into the full-scale street food operation that is Get It on a Bun at Booty's. Now *that's* the American Dream, folks.

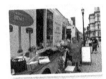

Tammy's menu is dominated by comfort food, but there's one thing she won't stand for—processed foods. She makes everything from scratch, and some of the ingredients even come from her own garden. Like many good food truck operators, she adjusts her menu seasonally, refreshing the crowd with a jalapeño-infused watermelon drink during the summer and helping them fight the chill with beans and cornbread when the temperatures begin to fall.

While I was chatting with Tammy, a customer walked up, squinting at the menu. "What's a booty dog?" he wanted to know.

Twenty minutes later he had an answer. "That was absolutely delicious," he said. "I'd make a special trip for that."

Here are two of Tammy's favorite recipes, no trip required: one for a true Southern classic—cornbread salad.

Tammy said, "This has always been my signature dish at holiday and family and friend gatherings. I've made this dish since the seventies. My dad loved it, and now I serve it out of my diner. He would be proud!"

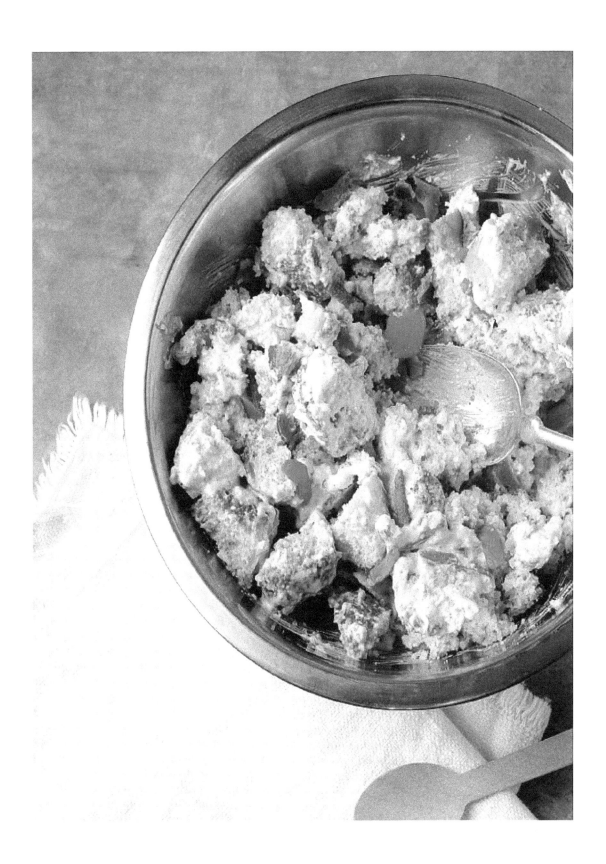

TAMMY'S CORNBREAD SALAD

Makes 12 servings.

Gather it up

3 boxes Jiffy cornbread mix, plus ingredients to make cornbread

½ cup pureed onion

6 hard-boiled eggs, finely diced

½ cup sweet pickle relish

1 (4-ounce) jar pimentos, drained

3 tablespoons yellow mustard

1 ½ cups mayonnaise

1 cup Miracle Whip

2 pounds hickory-smoked bacon, fried and crumbled

Salt and pepper to taste

Make it happen

Prepare the Jiffy cornbread according to the package directions and set aside to cool.

In a large bowl combine the onion, eggs, pickle relish, pimentos, mustard, mayonnaise, Miracle Whip, bacon, salt, and pepper. Mix until well blended. Break up the cooled cornbread and stir into the prepared dressing. Refrigerate overnight for the best flavor.

VEGGIE MELT

Makes 6 servings.

Gather it up

1 medium onion, thinly sliced

1 green bell pepper, sliced into strips

1 red bell pepper, sliced into strips

1 yellow bell pepper, sliced into strips

1 orange bell pepper, sliced into strips

¾ cup pickled banana pepper rings

2 tablespoons olive oil, plus more for the griddle

12 slices good-quality bread

6 slices Provolone cheese

6 slices American cheese

1 large ripe tomato, sliced

Celery salt to taste

Salt to taste

Black pepper to taste

Make it happen

Heat a large skillet over medium heat. Add the onions and peppers and sauté until the onions have softened.

Place the bread on a hot griddle or grill pan covered with olive oil. Place the slices of Provolone cheese on 6 slices of bread and the American cheese on the remaining 6 slices. Work in batches if needed. Place the sautéed veggies on the bread slices with celery salt, salt, pepper, and Provolone. Place a sliced tomato on top of the veggies. Flip the bread slices with the American cheese over the tomato, cheese side down. Continue flipping until golden brown on both sides and the cheese is melted.

Tammy says: "Cut the sandwich in half and see the beauty of all the colored peppers!"

GENIUS IN A BOX

LOUISVILLE

Concept: Gourmet sandwiches

mindspillinc.webs.com

Twitter: @giab8485

After months of saving for a wedding and a honeymoon, Tristian and Dierdre Barnes made a decision. There would be no wedding. Instead, they took the money they'd saved, bought a food truck, and headed to the courthouse for a no-frills vow swap. Someday they'll have that wedding; for now, they've got other goals. Like so many of their fellow food truckers, the Barneses got into the mobile dining game after being largely unfulfilled by traditional careers and the lack of jobs suited to their true interests. Tristian had nearly lost all patience with their situation one day while he and Dierdre were driving through the city. The couple happened to pass a food trailer on the side of the road with a For Sale sign on it. They doubled back, set up a time to meet with the owner, and Genius in a Box was born.

What should I order?

Give The Einstein a spin. You'll get a bagel bun filled with tender steak, two types of cheese, and sautéed onions.

"We're all geniuses in one way or another," Tristian told me, explaining the truck's unusual name. "This is just our way of recognizing that fact."

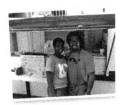

The Barneses decided to focus on sandwiches, dreaming up new ways to transform traditional ingredients into truly memorable lunches. English muffins, croissants, bagels, and potato buns stand in for regular bread, and they're not shy about piling on generous quantities of meats, cheeses, and veggies.

In keeping with the genius theme, each of the truck's sandwiches is named for a famous thinker. There's The Newton, which is an English muffin layered with Italian sausage, pepperoni, Colby and Cheddar cheeses, tomato, and romaine lettuce. Or The Plato, a grilled pork chop sandwich on a potato bun, dressed with cheese, tomato, and sautéed onions.

The ingredients are simple, but the finished product is pretty special.

THE RECIPE OF A GENIUS

Makes 6 servings.

Gather it up

1 tablespoon olive oil

1 red onion, thinly sliced into rings

1 green bell pepper, sliced into strips

1 pound Bavarian honey ham

1 pound hickory smoked bacon, cooked

1 (7-ounce) package pepperoni

6 slices Cheddar cheese

6 slices Pepper Jack cheese

6 potato bread buns, sliced

Make it happen

Heat the olive oil in a skillet over medium heat. Add the onions and green peppers and sauté until soft. Assemble the sandwiches by evenly dividing the ham, bacon, pepperoni, and Cheddar and Pepper Jack cheeses among the potato bread buns. Top each with the sautéed peppers and onions. Add any desired condiments and serve.

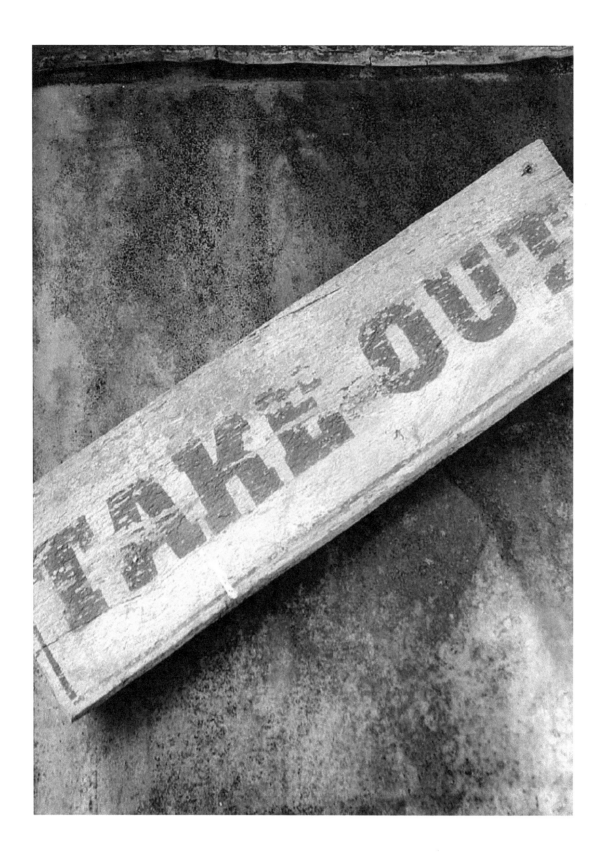

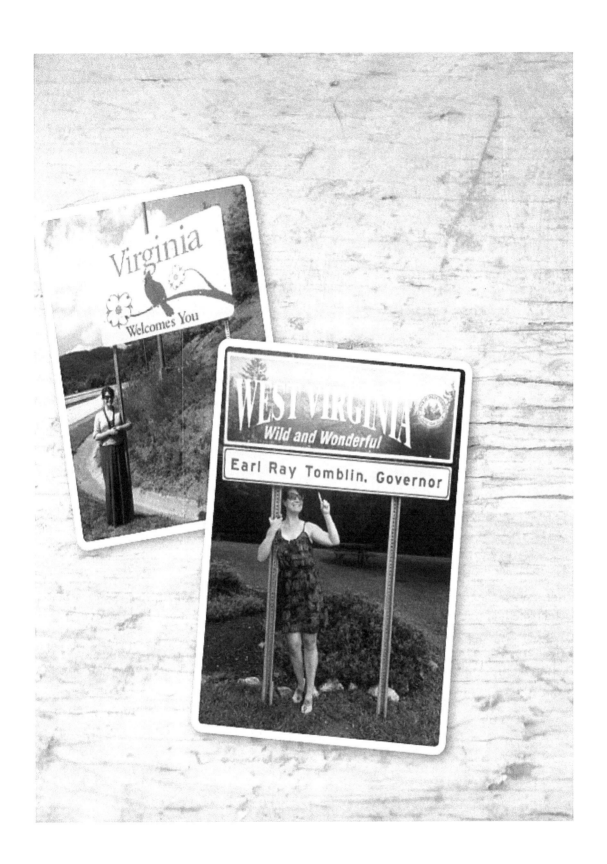

THE VIRGINIAS

Mission Savvy

Raw Thai Spring Rolls

Indonesian Curry

Vegan Tzatziki Sauce

BOKA Tako Truck

Red Curry Hummus

Glazed Apples

Dressed and Pressed

Grilled Lobster Tail Sandwich with Corn Relish and Tomato Vinaigrette

RVA Vegan

Potato Tacos

MISSION SAVVY

CHARLESTON, WEST VIRGINIA

Concept: Raw/Vegan

missionsavvy.com

 Facebook: facebook.com/MissionSavvyCafe

 Twitter: @MissionSavvyoTG

Jennifer Miller's presence alone is enough to make a person want to swear off fast food for good. That's the effect she had on me, at least. Lithe and luminous, Jennifer is poised in a way that seems nearly impossible, like a yoga instructor at some far-flung retreat by the ocean. But she doesn't live near any ocean, her home base being Charleston, West Virginia—that charming river city tucked amongst the Appalachian hills. In this beautiful, unlikely place, Jennifer runs Mission Savvy Juice Bar Cafe and Food Truck. It's a healthy dose of bright flavors and organic ingredients, devoted to introducing the region to raw and vegan cuisine in an unintimidating setting.

What should I order?

Go for the Sunshine Burger and a Carrot Orange Juice. The specials are sure-fire too.

"If you're not familiar with it, this is a lifestyle that can be a little overwhelming," Jennifer admits. "That's why I'm here. I want to make healthy eating more approachable."

Thanks to the culinary skill of Indira Riswanto, Mission Savvy's certified vegan chef, the menu delivers a delicious entry to a type of cuisine many people in Charleston may be trying for the first time.

"I had a fifty-year-old man come up to me at a festival we were working, and he said, 'My doctor says I need to cut out meat, but I don't know how to do that. What should I do?'" Jennifer recalled. "So I served him a veggie burger, and you know, he really liked it. Seeing somebody discover that for the first time is really exciting to me."

When she's not serving customers in her airy downtown café and boutique grocery store, Jennifer's on the road in her little Mission Savvy food truck, dishing up falafel burgers with vegan tzatziki, or watermelon juice, coconut water, and curry bowls—much of it raw, all of it vegan and delicious.

Not ready to go raw just yet? Baby-step it! Jennifer shared several recipes that serve as Exhibits A, B, C, and D of why a plant-based diet isn't as scary as you might think, and way more satisfying than you could have imagined.

RAW THAI SPRING ROLLS

Makes 10 rolls.

Gather it up

3 cups shredded carrots

3 cups chopped red bell pepper

1 cup chopped fresh mint

1 bunch cilantro, chopped

3 cups any kind of sprouts

10 sheets of rice paper

Almond Dipping Sauce (recipe follows)

Make it happen

Combine the carrots, red peppers, mint, cilantro, and sprouts in a large bowl. To assemble the rolls, spoon roughly one loose cup of the vegetable filling onto the end of each rice paper sheet. Fold the sides of the sheets inward over the vegetables, burrito-style, and then roll tightly toward you. If necessary, edges may be sealed with a small amount of water. Serve with Almond Dipping Sauce.

ALMOND DIPPING SAUCE

Makes 3 cups.

Gather it up

1 cup almond butter

1 tablespoon fresh lemon juice

½ tablespoon tamari sauce*

1 teaspoon sea salt

1 seeded jalapeño pepper

2 cups water

Make it happen

Add the almond butter, lemon juice, tamari sauce, sea salt, jalapeño, and water to the bowl of a food processor or blender and mix until creamy.

* Tamari sauce is a premium soy sauce that contains more soy and less wheat for a smoother taste.

INDONESIAN CURRY

Makes 6 servings.

Gather it up

1 cup diced onion

1 tablespoon minced garlic

2 cups broccoli florets

2 cups chopped carrots

4 cups peeled and cubed potatoes

2 cups green beans

1 tablespoon curry powder

2 teaspoons cumin

1 teaspoon sea salt, plus extra for seasoning

1 cup coconut milk

7 cups water

Make it happen

In a small nonstick pan over medium heat sauté the onion and garlic for 5 minutes until soft. Add the broccoli, carrots, potatoes, and green beans. Stir for 2 minutes. Add the curry, cumin, and salt, then stir for another 2 minutes. Pour the coconut milk and water into a large pot. Transfer the sautéed mixture to the pot and bring to a full boil over high heat. Reduce the heat to low and allow the vegetables to simmer for 10 to 15 minutes. Add extra salt to taste. Serve.

VEGAN TZATZIKI SAUCE

Makes 3 ½ cups.

Gather it up

2 cups almonds

5 cups water, divided

2 tablespoons fresh lemon juice

2 teaspoons salt

1 large cucumber, seeded and chopped

Make it happen

Soak the almonds in a bowl filled with 4 cups of water for 6 to 12 hours. Drain, rinse, and add the almonds to the bowl of a food processor. Add the lemon juice, salt, cucumber, and 1 cup water and blend until creamy. Can be used as a dip for veggies or pita.

BOKA TAKO TRUCK

RICHMOND, VIRGINIA

Concept: Asian-Mexican fusion

bokatruck.com

n facebook.com/pages/Boka-Tako-Truck

 Twitter: @BokaTruck

On the night I had planned to check out BOKA Tako Truck at Richmond's Hardywood Park Brewery, it was hot—summertime-in-the-South hot . . . 102 degrees at 6:00 p.m.—*that* kind of hot. To be honest, I really just wanted to retreat to my hotel room, where the AC was mercifully cranked to HI COOL. But I soldiered on, curious to see if BOKA would measure up to all the great things I'd read. I arrived at Hardywood to find several hundred Richmonders mixing around in the thick air, drinking icy craft brews, and lining up for paper trays of truck fare. The line at BOKA was a good twenty people deep. Here's a pro tip: always choose the food truck with the longest line. It'll be a wait that's well worth it.

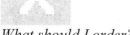

What should I order?

The Korean Beef Bulgogi Taco.

Technically, BOKA is a taco truck; but that's an oversimplification. While traditional Mexican street tacos (with a squeeze of lime, radishes, and Cotija cheese) will always be one of my favorite mobile meals, I appreciate the idea that you can put pretty much anything in a tortilla and achieve varying degrees of a favorable result. BOKA, run by Chef Patrick Harris, offers three taco styles: Mexican (Chihuahua cheese, habañero lime cabbage, and chipotle crema), Asian (sweet and spicy scratch-made kimchi, sesame aioli, and fresh herbs), and American (sherry slaw, smoky barbecue sauce, Jack and Cheddar cheeses, and caramelized onions). Any of these can be ordered with fish, beef, pork, or chicken. And just like any good food trucker does, Patrick nearly always has menu specials—his own inventive creations on display.

Perched low to the ground on a curb, I downed the Asian and Mexican iterations, along with an enchantingly memorable Shrimp and Grits Taco, which was stuffed with lots of crispy prosciutto and white Cheddar. The details at BOKA are what make it unforgettable. Each dish is festooned with some imaginative sauce, oil, aioli, or salsa. There's agave-marinated watermelon for the fish tacos, chili kraut for the kielbasa taco, and garlic confit for the butternut squash variety.

Chef Patrick shared up a couple of his favorite personal recipes here. If you're looking for a different way to enjoy hummus, you can't go wrong with this one. Give pita chips and baby carrots a break, and serve this one with thinly sliced radishes, sugar snap peas, and yellow bell peppers.

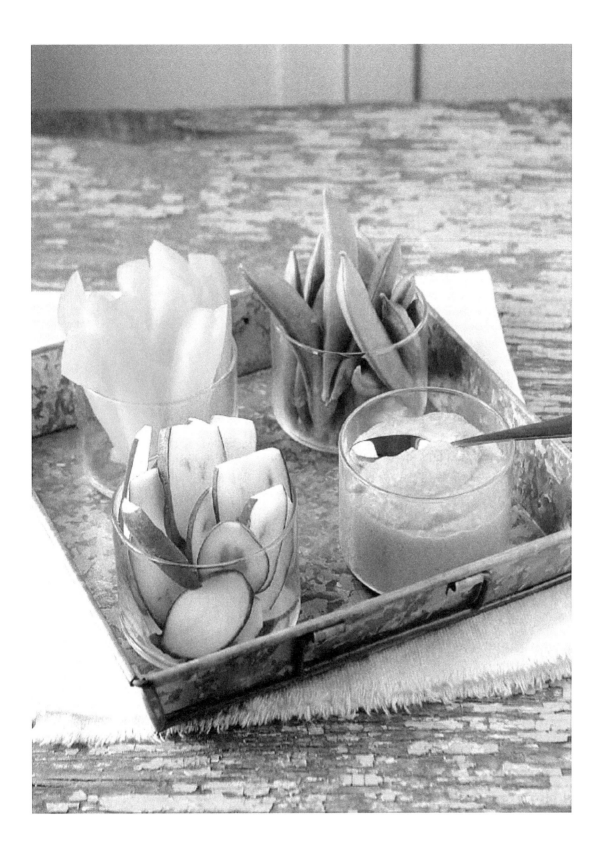

RED CURRY HUMMUS

Makes 2 cups.

Gather it up

2 (15-ounce) cans garbanzo beans

¾ cup tahini

Juice of 2 large lemons

3 tablespoons rice wine vinegar

1 tablespoon red curry

2 teaspoons minced garlic

1 teaspoon salt

1 ½ teaspoons sugar

2 teaspoons Sriracha

1 ½ teaspoons cumin

Make it happen

Drain half of the liquid from the beans and combine the beans, tahini, lemon juice, rice wine vinegar, red curry, garlic, salt, sugar, Sriracha, and cumin in the food processor. Process until ingredients are fully combined and the consistency takes on a smooth, almost whipped texture. Serve with your choice of cut veggies. Sliced radishes, sugar snap peas, and bell pepper strips work well.

GLAZED APPLES

Makes 12 servings.

Gather it up

10 Granny Smith apples, peeled, cored, and sliced

1 ½ cups butter, melted

¼ cup cider vinegar

2 tablespoons plus ½ teaspoon fresh lemon juice

8 whole cloves

¼ teaspoon pure ground allspice

2 cups sugar

1 teaspoon salt

½ tablespoon plus ½ teaspoon cinnamon

1 cup brown sugar

Make it happen

In a large pot combine the apples, butter, vinegar, lemon juice, cloves, allspice, sugar, salt, cinnamon, and brown sugar and bring to a boil over medium heat. Cook until the apples are tender. Remove the apples and cook the sauce until it thickens and forms a glaze. Return the apples to the pan and stir to combine.

DRESSED AND PRESSED

RICHMOND, VIRGINIA

Concept: Paninis and salads—all locally sourced and scratch-made.

DressedandPressed.com

 facebook.com/pages/Dressed-Pressed-gourmet-mobile-food-truck

Twitter: @DressedandPressed

This food truck took me to a place I never thought I'd find myself—an Indigo Girls concert. Despite *maybe* having owned one of their albums in college, I previously could not have imagined forking over the cash to see a live show.

After an unsuccessful attempt to catch up with Joe Andreoli and his Dressed and Pressed truck earlier in the day, I caught word through one of his street food peers that he had set up shop at the outdoor concert in beautiful Maymont Park (beautiful enough for a swing-by the next time you're in Richmond, by the way). Twenty minutes later I was chatting with Joe in the setting sunlight, laughing and straining to hear his story over the blaring chick rock. An hour later, I discovered that I really only needed to taste his story. While I stuffed my face with an order of Joe's famous truffle tots (they take twenty-four hours to prepare, start to finish!) and a Dressed Pork Po' Boy (fried pork on handmade ciabatta, pressed with crispy kale, pickles, mayo, mustard, and Cheddar), he told me about how his grandmother taught him to make her stunning but simple tomato sauce, how he spent a decade cheffing in some of the D.C.-area's top-tier restaurants (the venerable Inn at Little Washington in Virginia, to name just one), and how he holds his food truck to the same standards as any high-end brick-and-mortar establishment.

What should I order?

Whatever you order, order it with the truffle tots.

Joseph is devoted to sustainable agriculture, sourcing nearly everything on his menu from Virginia's abundance of area farms. "They're amazing," Joe told me, his face lighting up beneath a worn ball cap. "There are more than one hundred farms I could choose from at any given time. They're as fanatical about what they do as I am about what I do, so it really works out."

Joseph's willingness to share recipes is another thing that really works out. The next time you want to knock out a crowd, or maybe just your sweetie, make these lobster sandwiches. And that tomato vinaigrette? Feel free to drizzle liberally on pretty much anything you please. Fair warning: you may never buy bottled salad dressing again.

GRILLED LOBSTER TAIL SANDWICH WITH CORN RELISH AND TOMATO VINAIGRETTE

Makes 6 servings.

Gather it up

Vegetable or canola oil

3 lobster tails

½ cup (1 stick) butter, melted

½ cup mayonnaise

6 ciabatta rolls*

Corn Relish (recipe follows)

Tomato Vinaigrette (recipe follows)

Make it happen

Preheat the grill to medium heat and brush the grates with a little oil. Slice the lobster tails in half lengthwise and brush a small amount of oil onto the lobster flesh. Place the lobsters flesh side down for about 3 minutes, making sure there are no major flare-ups. Flip the lobsters over on the shell side and baste with butter. Repeat this step twice to achieve a rich, buttery flavor. Cook for about 3 minutes longer and remove from the heat.

Bring it all together

Spread some mayonnaise onto the bottom of the bread. Place a couple spoonfuls of the Corn Relish over the mayonnaise. After allowing the tail to cool for a few moments, slice width-wise, and arrange lobster pieces on top of the relish. Drizzle as much Tomato Vinaigrette onto the top piece of bread as desired and place on top of the lobster. Serve.

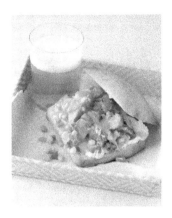

Available at most grocery store bakeries.

CORN RELISH

Makes 5 cups.

Gather it up

3 to 4 cups sweet corn, removed from cob

¼ cup diced red bell pepper

¼ cup diced green bell pepper

½ tablespoon seeded and minced jalapeño pepper

¼ cup diced red onion

2 tablespoons very finely chopped tarragon

¼ cup Tomato Vinaigrette (recipe follows)

Sugar to taste

Salt to taste

Black pepper to taste

Make it happen

Bring a large pot of water to a boil and add the corn kernels. Blanch until tender, 1 to 2 minutes, and drain. In a large bowl combine corn, bell peppers, jalapeño, red onion, tarragon, and Tomato Vinaigrette. Mix until combined. Add the sugar, salt, and pepper to taste.

TOMATO VINAIGRETTE

Makes 1 cup.

Gather it up

2 tomatoes, cored

4 tablespoons white balsamic vinegar

½ tablespoon tomato paste

3 tablespoons sour cream

½ tablespoon yellow mustard

½ cup extra virgin olive oil

1 teaspoon kosher salt

1 teaspoon sugar

Make it happen

In a blender or a food processor fitted with the blade attachment, combine the tomatoes, vinegar, tomato paste, sour cream, and mustard. Process until smooth. While the motor is running, add the extra virgin olive oil slowly, then add salt and sugar. Allow to process for a minute or so until emulsified. Slowly pour through a fine mesh strainer.

RVA VEGAN

RICHMOND, VIRGINIA

Concept: Vegan cupcakes and tacos

www.rvavegan.info

 facebook.com/pages/RVA-Vegan

Twitter: @veganrva

In a moment of startling honesty, Ed Edge—a fourteen-year vegan—admitted something to me. "I don't even really like vegan food that much," he said. "Most of what's out there just doesn't grab me."

That's why his approach with RVA Vegan is pretty different from the average kale-and-quinoa vegan scene. Admittedly, his menu is kind of random—tacos, po' boys, hot dogs, tamales, and cupcakes. He cops to having "positively no culinary background whatsoever," except for knowing what he likes to eat. But a single bite of an RVA cupcake (triple chocolate! caramel maple! fruit punch!) is all you really need to understand that "formal education" can sometimes be way overrated.

What should I order?

Mandarin Chocolate Cupcake

"I just make food that tastes good," Ed explained. "It may not be very fancy, but the fact of the matter is that 99 percent of my customers aren't even vegetarian. The only way they're going to look at vegan food is if it's as close to 'normal' food as possible."

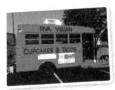

Ed agreed to part with the recipe for his Potato Taco, one of the most popular items on the RVA Vegan menu. You'd be wise to keep these ingredients on hand at all times. This is the perfect flavor-packed recipe that requires virtually no prep. Just heat everything in a pan, spoon it into your tortillas, and dinner is done. You won't believe how delicious it is until you try it.

Ed says: I was going to send a more ornate recipe, but they can be awfully discouraging and involve hard-to-find ingredients. This is simple, cheap, and satisfying.

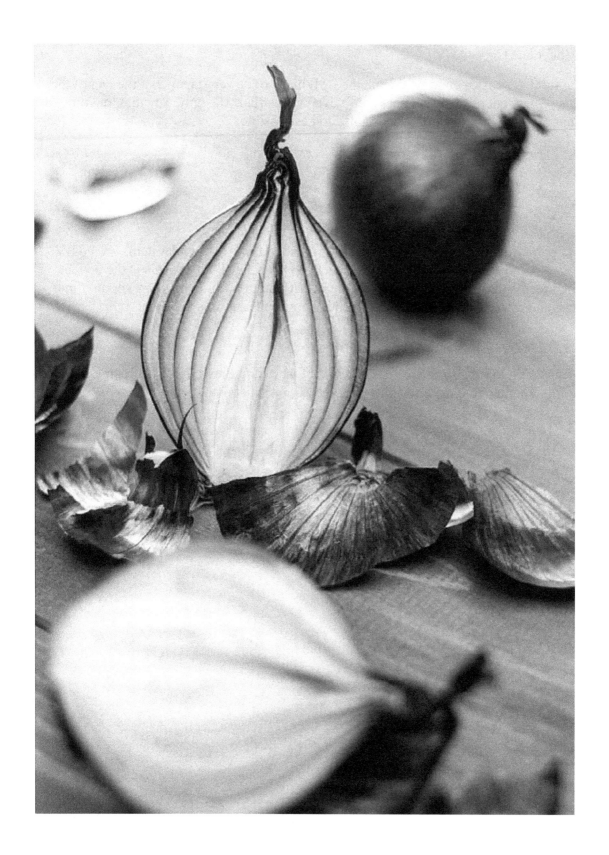

POTATO TACOS

Makes 16 tacos.

Gather it up

1 tablespoon butter-flavored vegetable oil spread

3 cans diced white potatoes

1 red onion, diced

1 tablespoon paprika

1 tablespoon ground red pepper

1 tablespoon Sriracha sauce

2 (10-ounce) cans Rotel tomato and jalapeño mix

1 (15-ounce) can black beans

1 (14-ounce) can white corn

16 small flour tortillas

Make it happen

Melt the vegetable oil spread in a large skillet over medium heat. Add the potatoes, onions, paprika, red pepper, and Sriracha sauce to the skillet. Stir everything until mixed thoroughly and the potatoes are orange. Allow to cook for 3 minutes. Drain the Rotel, black beans, and white corn, and add to the skillet. Mix thoroughly, cover the skillet, and cook 3 to 5 minutes until heated through. Divide the mixture evenly among tortillas, fold in half, and serve.

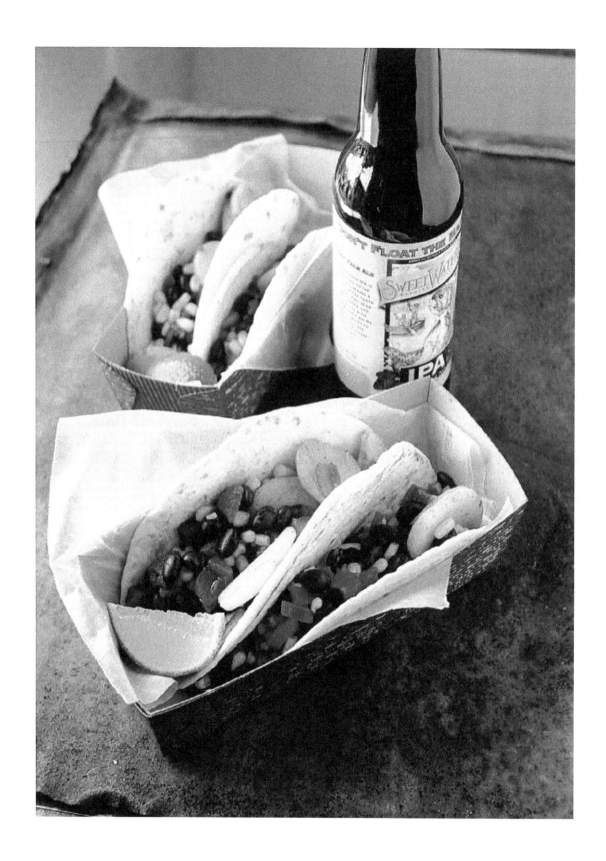

NORTH CAROLINA

Triangle Raw Foods

TRF Pad Thai

TRF Chocolate Tarts

Porchetta

Basil Pork Sausage

Basil Pesto

Chirba Chirba

Chirba Chive Dumplings

Roaming Fork

Fried Deviled Eggs

The Tin Kitchen

Cilantro-Lime Aioli

Green Rice

Pineapple Pico de Gallo

Big Mike's BBQ

Blue Cheese Cole Slaw

Big Mike's Mac 'n' Cheese

TRIANGLE RAW FOODS

RALEIGH-DURHAM

Concept: Raw food

trianglerawfoods.com

 facebook.com/Triangle.Raw.Foodists

Twitter: @TriangleRawFood

I've come to really love the unexpected. When you tell somebody you're writing a cookbook about food trucks in the Southeast, the assumption can be that you're writing a book full of barbecue, macaroni, and biscuit recipes. And while this book certainly features some bang-up versions of those dishes, there are also some surprises—Triangle Raw Foods, for one. Jane Howard Crutchfield and Matthew Daniels had their softly lit food cart stationed outside of Durham's Fullsteam Brewery when I caught up with them during a lightning storm on a Friday night. Muggy air, microbrews, and a couple of fresh-scrubbed raw foodists giving me the lowdown on how they happily sustain and share their lifestyle in the meat-adoring South—it was all pretty perfect. But Jane and Matthew didn't just tell me their story; they *showed* me. I feasted on a sweet potato apple salad with maple-black pepper vinaigrette, Asian marinated kale, and a bafflingly flavorful pad thai.

What should I order?

The pad thai. Definitely the pad thai. Who knew pad thai without noodles was even possible?

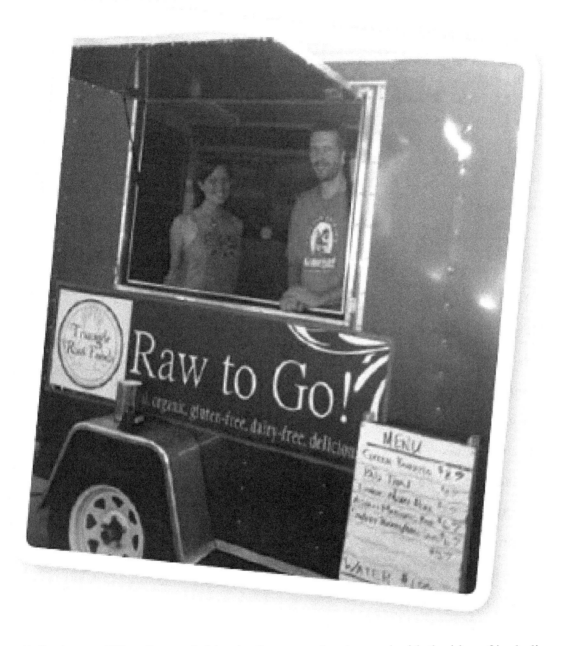

Full disclosure: When I started this trip, I was nearly obsessed with the idea of including a few vegan and raw food trucks. While I am neither a vegan nor a raw foodist, I am fascinated by people who are.

Jane and Matthew were vegan for years before they tried the raw route, loved how great they felt, and never went back! There was only one problem: Durham can be a challenging place for a raw foodist. The couple realized that if they wanted to eat anything more than regular salads at restaurants, they'd have to make it themselves.

If you hear the words *vegan* or *raw* and automatically stop listening, then you need to back up and reconsider. Remember: you don't have to *be* a raw foodist to try or even enjoy raw cuisine. It's fresh, it's teeming with flavor, and it's so, so, so good for you. Try it, and see what Jane and Matthew have known all along.

I'll be honest. We're all pretty lucky that I was able to snag Triangle Raw Foods' recipe for that glorious pad thai. If I were to make a list of the top five recipes in this book that you *need* to make, this would certainly be on the list. Try it for yourself, and marvel at how zucchini can magically stand in for noodles.

TRF PAD THAI

Makes 4 to 6 servings.

Gather it up

5 medium to large zucchinis, spiralized*

2 carrots, shredded

2 Thai chiles (or more if you want more heat)

2 garlic cloves

4 sun-dried tomatoes, reconstituted**

½ cup sesame oil

¼ cup tamari or soy sauce

3 tablespoons tamarind paste

2 tablespoons chili powder

1 tablespoon paprika

1 tablespoon mirin

1 teaspoon fresh lime juice

⅓ cup chopped cilantro, for garnish

¼ cup crushed raw cashews, for garnish

Lime slices, for garnish

Make it happen

In a large bowl mix the spiralized zucchini and shredded carrots until evenly distributed.

In a food processor using the S blade, pulse the Thai chiles, garlic, and sun-dried tomatoes until minced. Add the sesame oil, tamari, tamarind paste, chili powder, paprika, mirin, and lime juice and process for about 1 minute on high speed.

Pour the sauce over the zucchini and carrots and mix until well-coated. Garnish with cilantro, cashews, and a slice of lime.

* Jane and Matthew recommend using a Paderno World Cuisine Spiral Vegetable Slicer (available on Amazon.com, but check your local kitchen store first). You can also use a mandoline or a julienne peeler.

** To reconstitute, soak in water for at least an hour.

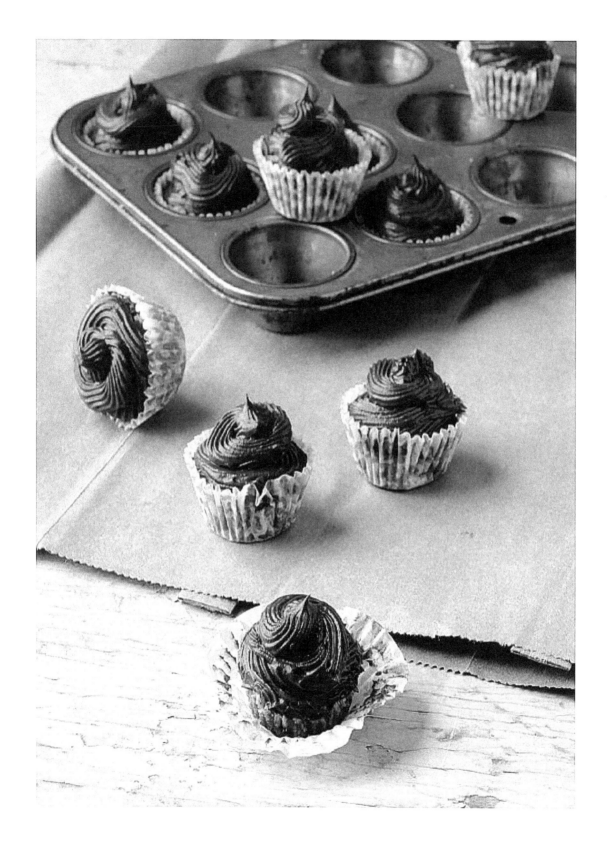

TRF CHOCOLATE TARTS

Makes 12 mini tarts.

Gather it up

1 cup raw walnuts, soaked and dehydrated

1 cup raw pecans, soaked and dehydrated

6 medjool dates

2 ripe avocados

¼ cup pure maple syrup

¼ cup raw cacao powder (use more for darker chocolate)

1 teaspoon ground vanilla bean

Make it happen

To make the crust: Place the walnuts, pecans, and dates in the bowl of a food processor. Pulse until it becomes a dough-like consistency. Line a mini muffin tin with mini muffin wrappers. With your fingers or a spoon, press 1 ½ tablespoons of nut mixture into each wrapper for the tart crust.

To make the filling: Slice the avocados in half and remove the pit. Scoop out the pulp and place in the bowl of a food processor equipped with the S blade. Add maple syrup, cacao, and vanilla and process until the ingredients reach a creamy consistency. Spoon the mixture on top of the tart crusts (or you can use a piping bag) and enjoy.

PORCHETTA

RALEIGH-DURHAM

Concept: Italian-style pork

porchettardu.com

 facebook.com/Porchettardu

Twitter: @Porchettardu

What do trained chefs joke about? Owning a food truck, of course! Every once in a while, the joke simmers down, and they find themselves wondering, *Well, actually . . . what if?* That's pretty much how everything unfolded for Nicholas Crosson and Matthew Hayden when they met in the kitchen at 18 Seaboard, one of the most celebrated restaurants in Raleigh, known for its inventive takes on American classics and focus on locally sourced ingredients. Crosson, who attended culinary school in France and spent considerable time in Italy and Spain, loved the idea of bridging the gap between North Carolina's dining sensibilities and the flavors and techniques he discovered in Europe. The foundation of Nicholas and Matthew's operation is pork, specifically its namesake, porchetta—a pork roast wrapped in pork belly and filled with herbs and spices. After a long, slow roast, the meat is shaved into savory shreds of porky goodness.

You might think of it as the Italians' answer to the pulled pork we Southerners love so dearly. The Porchetta guys pile that tender, herby meat high on Kaiser rolls and let the customers choose where to take it from there. You can add Provolone and grainy mustard, or pickled hot peppers and sweet pepper chutney, or roasted tomato and basil pesto, among other options.

What should I order?

Starting with The Original might be the obvious advice, but why not take the plunge and order The Mediterranean? You'll get a Kaiser roll towering with shaved Italian-style pork, roasted red peppers, caramelized onions, mozzarella cheese, and herb aioli.

If you can tear yourself away from the marquee attraction, you might try one of Porchetta's handmade pork and lamb sausages, pork burgers, or salads. Nicholas and Matthew buy their heritage-grade hogs through the North Carolina Natural Hog Growers Association, an organization of farmers who raise their pigs under slightly stricter standards than organic labeling requirements. This allows Porchetta to partner with small farms throughout the state, support the local economy, and buy top-quality hogs that yield the best culinary outcome.

Porchetta may have started as a joke, but it's shaping up to be one of the best ideas to hit the Triangle's food truck scene.

BASIL PORK SAUSAGE

Makes 5 pounds.

EQUIPMENT NOTE: *This recipe requires a meat grinder or a stand mixer with a meat grinder attachment and a sausage stuffing tube.*

Gather it up

3 ½ pounds lean pork shoulder

1 pound pork fat back

½ cup chopped fresh garlic

⅓ cup fresh basil

3 tablespoons kosher salt

6 feet of pork casings

Make it happen

Dice the pork shoulder and cube the fat back into ½-inch pieces, removing as much of the sinew and silver skin as you can. Combine the two in a large bowl. Add the chopped garlic to the bowl. Chop the basil and add it to the bowl as well. Add the salt and toss to coat, creating an even mixture. Place the bowl in the freezer for 20 minutes to ensure the meat grinds more easily.

Attach your grinder attachment to your stand mixer according to manufacturer's specifications and use a medium-size die. Feed the pork mixture through the grinder. If you notice the fat starting to run, place the bowl and the attachment in the freezer for 10 minutes. After all the meat has been ground, place the bowl in the fridge for 30 minutes.

Attach your sausage stuffing tube to the meat grinding attachment on the stand mixer and pull the casing over the tube.* Pinch the end of the casing and feed the meat into the hopper. The meat will feed into the casing, and as it does, try to ensure an even fill. Also, make sure not to overfill, as this will cause the casing to rip when you pinch and twist the sausage into links.

After all the casings have been filled, pinch off the sausage to your desired size and twist each sausage in alternating directions. Refrigerate for at least 4 hours before cutting the links apart.

To prepare, boil the sausage for 10 minutes and then brown in a skillet for best taste and texture.

There are great tutorials on YouTube if you need a good visual.

BASIL PESTO

Makes 1 ½ cups.

Gather it up

1 cup fresh basil

½ cup fresh curly parsley

1 garlic clove

Juice of ½ lemon

¼ cup shaved Parmesan cheese

¼ cup toasted pine nuts

⅛ teaspoon salt

½ cup olive oil

Make it happen

Rough chop the basil, parsley, and garlic and place in the bowl of a food processor. Add the lemon juice, cheese, pine nuts, salt, and olive oil and process until all the ingredients have just come together, leaving some texture. If the mixture will not blend, add just a touch more oil until it does. This makes an excellent accompaniment to the Basil Pork Sausage.

CHIRBA CHIRBA

DURHAM

Concept: Chinese-style dumplings

chirbachirba.com

 facebook.com/chirbachirba

 Twitter: @chirbachirba

Let's pretend your home has always been beautiful North Carolina. In such a scenario, you know the difference between Eastern- and Western-style barbecue sauce. You refuse to acknowledge any jar of mayonnaise that doesn't carry the Duke's label. And you hold firm that the best soft drink with a red and white label is Cheerwine, of course. And then let's pretend that you move far away. To China, perhaps? There's no Cheerwine there, and no smoky pulled pork doused in Carolina barbecue sauce. And then it happens. You start to miss the flavors of home.

What should I order?

Porkedame dumplings, filled with pork, scallions, and edamame.

Well, flip the script, and that's exactly the situation Chela Tu and several of her fellow Chinese classmates found themselves in while they were undergraduates at the University of North Carolina, Chapel Hill. "We had a strong passion for recreating the things from home that we loved, but couldn't easily find around here," Chela said. "I started hosting dumpling-making parties at my apartment, because that was one thing we all missed. At some point we realized the potential in what we were doing."

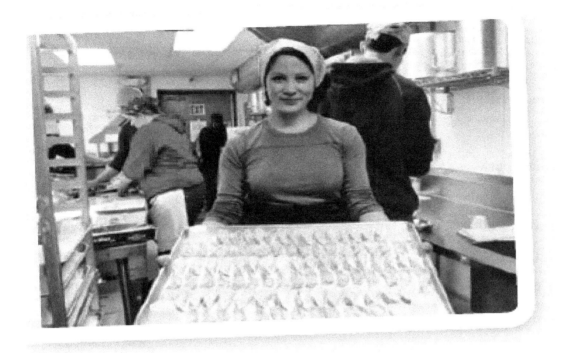

And that was the beginning for Chirba Chirba, which essentially translates to "Eat Eat" in English. Chela's three partners, Yin Song, Nate Adams, and Ali Safavi, realized their Chinese-style dumplings could easily be sold and enjoyed as street food in the Raleigh-Durham-Chapel Hill Triangle. So they pooled their knowledge, finances, experience, and connections to transform an old taco truck into a bright yellow dumpling-mobile.

Chirba Chirba's dumplings—little pouches of dough filled with meat, veggies, and spices before being boiled, steamed, or fried—became an instant hit in the Triangle and beyond. In 2012, the Chirba Chirba gang even found themselves featured on an episode of the LiveWell Network show "My Family Recipe Rocks," where they shared their story and the secrets to their dumpling magic. As for the secret to their success, Chela believes it has everything to do with their initial approach.

"We took every aspect of this idea seriously," she said. "We had a really good business plan, and we thought out every last detail thoroughly. We were serious about how we were going to pay for the business, how we were going to make the dumplings delicious, how we were going to get people to buy them. We didn't leave anything to chance."

Chela's letting us all in on another secret: the recipe for the Chirba Chive Dumplings. She strongly suggests you make a party of it! Set aside an evening, invite some friends over, and take on the challenge of assembling delicious pork dumplings.

CHIRBA CHIVE DUMPLINGS

Gather it up

Special equipment:

Chopsticks

Bamboo steamer basket

½ pound ground pork

4 ½ tablespoons vegetable oil

4 teaspoons sesame oil

4 teaspoons soy sauce

4 teaspoons mushroom soy sauce

¼ teaspoon sugar

½ teaspoon salt

½ teaspoon white pepper

1 teaspoon ground ginger

3 tablespoons potato starch

½ cup Chinese celery, chopped*

¾ cup Chinese chives, chopped*

¼ cup scallions

1 package dumpling wrappers*

1 head Napa cabbage

Black Chinese vinegar, for serving*

Make it happen

Combine the pork, vegetable and sesame oils, and regular and mushroom soy sauces in a large bowl and mix well. Add the sugar, salt, pepper, ginger, and potato starch and mix well. Add the celery, chives, and scallions and thoroughly combine into the meat mixture. Make sure the scallions are the last addition, as the onions can contribute a slimy texture when marinating in the meat for too long. Now, go wake up your dough!

Grab some friends. A dumpling-making party is big fun for a group (that is how Chirba Chirba began, after all). Assign some people to pleat and one to boil/steam!

Place a spoonful of filling (start small and work your way up—less filling is easier to pleat) in the center of your wrapper. Here, you've got form and function to consider. The function of your pleat should be to seal the meat inside the wrapper so that no filling can escape during the cooking process. You can do this simply by folding the wrapper over the filling in a half-circle shape and pinching the edges closed. You'll need a little dish of water to wet the edges in order for the wrapper to stick to itself around the filling.

The idea behind the pleating process (the form) is to make the dumpling pretty with various pleats and folds. To do this, fold your wrapper in half around the meat and pinch it on the top. It looks like a taco but sealed at one point at the top. Place the taco round side up on your index finger that should be hook shaped pointing sideways and hold it steady with your thumb (that has the same curvature as your index finger). Now bring your other hand on the other side of the taco and press the edges of the dumpling against your curved index finger with your two thumbs. The positioning of your thumbs around the edge of the dumplings will feel very awkward at first, but you'll get used to it. If you don't curve your thumbs, then you'll just end up squeezing the meat filling out of the sides and then you'll have to start over.

Don't be discouraged; practice makes perfect! You can find lots of helpful videos online with different pleating techniques.

To steam: Prepare a bamboo steamer basket over a saucepan of boiling water. Make sure the water doesn't touch the bottom of the basket. Line the basket with Napa cabbage leaves and place 7 to 8 dumplings at a time on top of the cabbage. Steam the dumplings for 10 minutes.

To boil: Bring a large pot of water to a rolling boil over high heat. Drop half of the dumplings into the boiling water. When the water returns to a boil, add a cup of cold water. Repeat two more times. Serve with black Chinese vinegar.

* All these products are available at Asian grocery stores.

Note: Chinese celery is thin stalked and has a stronger flavor than traditional celery sold in grocery stores. Feel free to substitute regular celery in a pinch.

ROAMING FORK

CHARLOTTE

Concept: Eclectic Southern

roamingfork.net

◼ facebook.com/pages/Roaming-Fork

Twitter: @roamingforkNC

When Kelli Crisan moved to Charlotte from Orlando several years ago, she kept wondering, *Where are the food carts?* She was accustomed to perusing Florida's bustling mobile food scene for a terrific selection of eats, and she couldn't believe the trend hadn't found its way to Charlotte. So she dreamt up Roaming Fork and expedited the process herself. Kelli envisioned a food truck menu full of items that make you do a double take when you see them. Delights such as a three-cheese pulled pork grilled cheese sandwich on crispy sourdough, fried deviled eggs, and truffle Parmesan fries (voted the best fries in Charlotte!) dominate the Roaming Fork menu, which is a fixture at Charlotte-area festivals, office parks, and curbsides. Almost two years in, the city can't seem to get enough of Kelli's creations—especially her blackened fish tacos, which are often served with a zesty mango salsa.

What should I order?

The blackened fish tacos are a rightfully popular mainstay, but if the smoked meatloaf sandwich is on the menu while you're there, go for that.

Despite Roaming Fork's menu full of Southern flair, there was definitely a breaking-in period for people who didn't know what the heck to think of a food truck. "There was some education that had to happen, definitely," Kelli said. "But people here have been quick learners. Once they take a look at the menu, they're drawn in."

If you're still thinking about those fried deviled eggs Kelli serves, then you're going to like the recipe she shared here. Whip up a batch of these golden brown beauties next time you're invited to a backyard barbecue. They're salty, tangy, crunchy, and sure to get you invited over again.

You can thank Kelli the next time you're in Charlotte!

FRIED DEVILED EGGS

Makes 10–12 servings.

Gather it up

1 dozen eggs (local, if possible), hard-boiled and cooled

1 scallion, white and green parts, finely diced

¼ red onion, finely diced

4 slices applewood smoked bacon strips, cooked crisp and crumbled

⅓ cup shredded sharp Cheddar cheese

1 teaspoon smoked Hungarian paprika

Garlic powder to taste

Salt and black pepper to taste

1 tablespoon Dijon mustard

½ cup mayonnaise*

1 ½ cups flour (mix with a dash or two of paprika for extra flavor)

1 cup buttermilk

1 ½ cups panko bread crumbs

Vegetable oil for frying

Honey mustard dipping sauce, for serving

Make it happen

Place the cooled, hard-boiled eggs in a food processor and pulse enough to chop them up but not enough to make them mushy. Place in a large bowl and add the scallion, red onion, bacon, cheese, paprika, garlic powder, salt, and pepper. Mix all ingredients well with your hands, then add the Dijon mustard and mayonnaise. You can always add more mustard and mayonnaise if needed, but you don't want an overly wet mixture.

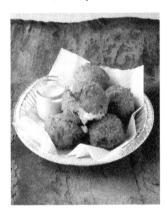

Once everything is blended, shape the mixture into 10 to 12 Ping-Pong ball–size egg shapes, and place in the freezer for about 30 minutes, or long enough to firm them up. This makes the handling process for dipping and frying much easier.

While the eggs are in the freezer, prepare three pans (pie plates work well): one with flour, one with buttermilk, and one with the panko bread crumbs. Preheat a deep-fryer or deep skillet with oil heated to 350 degrees.

Dredge each of the firmed-up eggs once in each pie plate: flour, buttermilk, panko—in that order—and gently place in the hot oil. Fry until the outside is golden brown. Remove from the oil, sprinkle with a dash of salt, and serve with your favorite honey mustard dipping sauce.

* *Use Duke's brand, if available.*

THE TIN KITCHEN

CHARLOTTE

Concept: Gourmet Tacos

thetinkitchen.com

 facebook.com/TheTINKitchen

Twitter: @TheTINKitchen

When I met up with the guys of the Tin Kitchen, their truck was parked at an event that never actually happened. I believe it was an outdoor movie night. The scrawny crowd was bad for business, but it worked out pretty great for me. Over the course of two hours, Team Tin Kitchen—Chef David Stuck, Chef Charlie Reid, and their business partner, Nick Lischerong—traded zingers, talked shop about culinary school, and prepared everything on their menu for me to try. *Everything.* I dined on pork belly tacos with kimchi and hoisin glaze, smoked salmon tacos smothered in pineapple pico de gallo (recipe follows!), BBQ brisket tacos with chipotle slaw and shaved scallions, and veggie tacos filled with sweet potato hash, white beans, and goat cheese. It was the remarkable sort of spread you'd expect from a couple of trained chefs who've worked in top-tier restaurant kitchens all over the east and west coasts.

What should I order?

The BBQ Brisket Tacos, of course!

Somewhere in the mix, Charlie handed me a small paper cup filled with something he innocently called "pickled veg." Looking back, he may have mentioned something about heat and to be careful. And looking back, I may have waved him off and mentioned something about having a "high tolerance" for heat. I do remember being very cavalier about it, tipping back the cup for a huge mouthful, and chomping down confidently. And I remember my mouth, throat, sinuses, and ear canals catching fire as I sat in the front seat of the Tin Kitchen. Attempts to douse the flames with my drink came up short. My eyes spilled over with heat-tears. My nose started to run. I couldn't talk. For a few minutes, the guys were blessedly occupied with something on the grill, and I thought for sure I could get it under control before they called my bluff. But I couldn't. They laughed, and I lost whatever shred of foodie cred I may have had with these guys.

Fortunately, they didn't hold it against me. They sent me the recipes for this terrific trio of accompaniments they serve with several of their tacos on the truck. My advice to you, dear reader: try these recipes for a flavor upgrade on your next taco night. No bluffing necessary!

CILANTRO-LIME AIOLI

Makes 1 ½ cups.

Gather it up

1 cup mayonnaise

½ cup fresh lime juice

2 bunches cilantro, washed and stalks removed

½ cup fresh spinach

1 cup kosher salt

¼ cup black pepper

Make it happen

Combine the mayonnaise, lime juice, cilantro, spinach, salt, and pepper in a blender or food processor and puree until smooth. Refrigerate.

GREEN RICE

Makes 12 servings.

Gather it up

2 bunches cilantro, chopped

3 jalapeño peppers, seeded and sliced

9 scallions, sliced

4 garlic cloves, chopped

3 cups fresh spinach

6 tablespoons butter

3 tablespoons fresh lime juice

3 tablespoons kosher salt

1 tablespoon black pepper

10 ½ cups hot water

6 ¾ cups parboiled* rice

Make it happen

Preheat the oven to 450 degrees.

In a blender, combine the cilantro, jalapeños, scallions, garlic, spinach, butter, lime juice, salt, pepper, and water, and blend until smooth. Put the rice in a large baking pan and pour the mixture over the rice. Bake for 35 minutes.

* Parboiled rice is partially cooked, often found in microwavable packages.

PINEAPPLE PICO DE GALLO

Makes about 6 cups.

Gather it up

5 cups pineapple chunks

2 jalapeño peppers, seeded and minced

¾ bunch cilantro, chopped

½ red onion, diced

Juice of 3 limes

1 teaspoon black pepper

1 teaspoon kosher salt

Make it happen

In a large bowl combine the pineapple, jalapeños, cilantro, onion, lime juice, pepper, and salt and mix well. Chill in the refrigerator for a few hours and serve.

BIG MIKE'S BBQ

RALEIGH-DURHAM

CONCEPT: Smoked meats and Southern sides

apexbbq.com

◼ facebook.com/pages/Big-Mikes-BBQ

  Twitter: @bigmikesbbqnc

East to West

North Carolina is full of choices: Duke or UNC, mountains or coast, eastern vs. western barbecue sauce. Here's a little sauce primer for the uninitiated:

Eastern-style: a vinegar-based sauce made with a mild vinegar and water and flavored with hot peppers, black pepper, and white sugar.

Western-style: also a vinegar-based sauce but with the addition of a tomato component (paste, puree, or ketchup) along with spices and brown sugar. This is also sometimes referred to as "Lexington style."

A lot of smack-talk about barbecue gets traded around in the South, especially in North Carolina. Whether the pig is chopped, blocked, pulled, or slathered in Eastern or Western North Carolina-style sauce, nearly every meat eater in the state has an opinion. Michael Markham certainly did. While restaurants that serve barbecue aren't scarce in the Triangle, everything he tried fell short of his expectations. So he quit his complaining and did something about it. He started his own mobile dining and catering business. Michael had always enjoyed cooking and was no stranger to a meat smoker, so the plunge felt pretty natural. Alongside his smoked ribs, pulled pork, brisket, turkey, and sausage, Michael offers up a slew of side dishes. When I dined at Big Mike's, he hooked me up with a big pile of brisket, a serving of blue cheese coleslaw, a heaping helping of macaroni and cheese, and his signature brisket-studded baked beans. Now, I'm pretty well acquainted with the smoked meat/coleslaw/macaroni/baked bean scene. I've eaten my share of those foods, but Big Mike's renditions of these Southern standards are truly remarkable. Also impressive? The Big Mike's BBQ rig itself! Michael serves his fare out of a miniature red barn, complete with a screen porch and an on-board smoker.

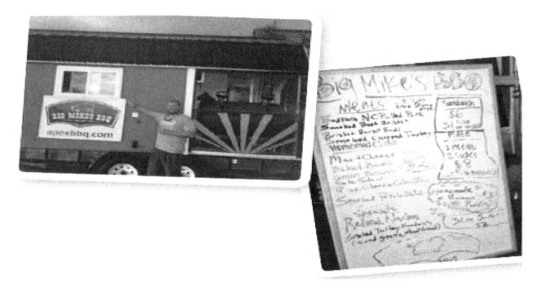

What should I order?

Hands-down, the brisket burnt ends (trust me) and the macaroni and cheese.

Yes, there's lots of barbecue in North Carolina, but Big Mike's is worth your time. And if at the end of your meal you still have some room left, don't miss out on Michael's homemade banana pudding—with bacon or without. My advice: with! If pudding's not your thing, grab one of the handmade oatmeal cream pies or a cinnamon sugar pretzel with buttercream icing!

In the meantime, try your hand at a couple of Michael's most popular menu items.

BLUE CHEESE COLESLAW

Makes 6 servings.

Gather it up

¾ cup sour cream

¼ cup mayonnaise

¼ cup white balsamic vinegar

Salt and black pepper to taste

½ head green cabbage, thinly shredded

2 carrots, washed, peeled, and shredded

½ cup blue cheese crumbles

Make it happen

In a large bowl blend the sour cream, mayonnaise, and vinegar until smooth. Add salt and pepper to taste. Fold in the cabbage, carrots, and blue cheese crumbles, and stir gently to combine. Refrigerate.

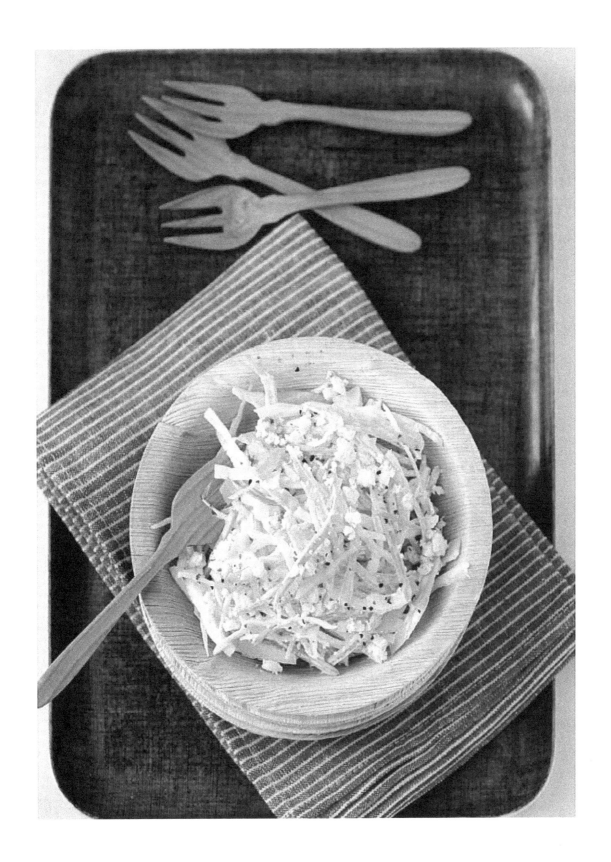

BIG MIKE'S MAC 'N' CHEESE

Makes 6 to 8 servings.

Gather it up

1 pound elbow macaroni, cooked and drained

¼ cup butter, melted

1 egg

1 (8-ounce) can evaporated milk

2 teaspoons dry mustard

1 tablespoon hot sauce

½ cup whole milk

1 cup white Cheddar cheese (the sharper, the better), plus extra for topping

Salt and black pepper to taste

Make it happen

Preheat the oven to 350 degrees. Grease a 9 × 13-inch casserole dish.

In a large bowl combine the macaroni, butter, egg, evaporated milk, dry mustard, hot sauce, milk, cheese, salt, and pepper. Mix well and pour into the casserole dish and bake uncovered for 20 minutes. Add extra cheese and place under the broiler for a few minutes for a golden brown crust.

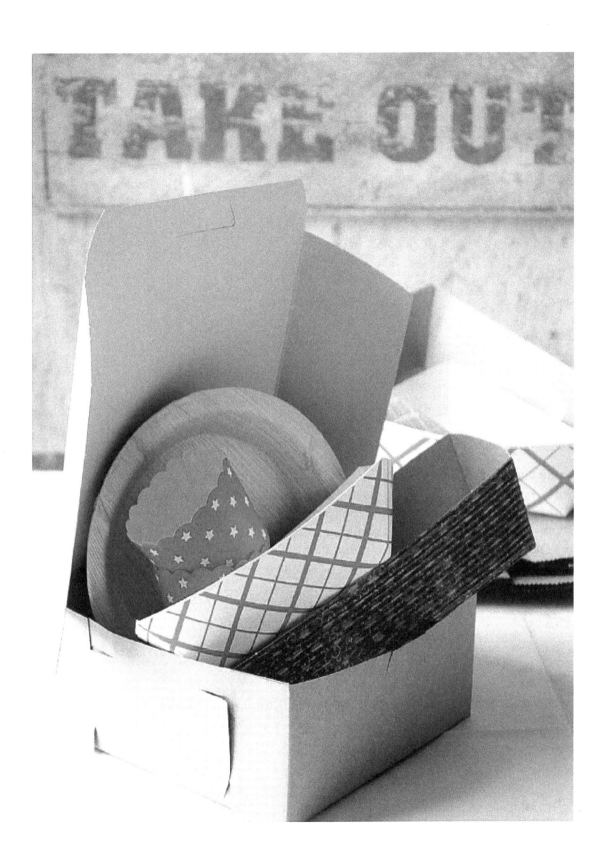

SOUTH CAROLINA

Foodie Truck

Foodie Truck's Shepherd's Pie

Dulce Truck

Double-Layer Chocolate Cake

Peach Spice Sweet Tea

Cast Iron Grill

Mad Cap Portobello Mushroom Sandwich

FOODIE TRUCK

CHARLESTON

Concept: Street gourmet

foodietruck.net

 facebook.com/FoodieTruck

 Twitter: @FoodieTruck

Jonathan Corey and Jon Amato are old culinary school pals. After graduating from Johnson & Wales in Norfolk, Virginia, in 2004, they went their separate ways—Jonathan to the Virgin Islands, Jon to Washington D.C. The pair reconnected in Charleston, where they found themselves working in two of the city's acclaimed restaurant kitchens—McCrady's and FIG, respectively. They bonded over the idea of striking out on their own, building a food truck that wouldn't require their loyalty to any one particular menu concept.

What should I order?

The Picnic Biscuit: a Cheddar biscuit stuffed with pork confit, preserved tomato, and Dijon mustard.

They wanted to do it all . . . and they do. American, Asian fusion, seafood, Italian, Mexican, Southern comfort—the Foodie Truck menu dabbles in so very many flavor profiles. Steamed buns filled with Korean barbecue and crunchy veggies share truck space with a fried green tomato BLT on jalapeño cornbread. And in what seems to be one of Foodie Truck's most obvious crowd favorites, Jon and Jonathan serve a Philly cheesesteak gussied up with pickled green tomatoes, fried salami, and a special "truck blend" sauce.

"We wanted a modern restaurant approach to the truck food that included fresh seasonal ingredients," Jonathan said. "We wanted to be able to serve whatever struck a chord with us—

tacos, banh mi, dumplings—rather than ourselves to one genre." And Charleston has responded overwhelmingly to the concept. "It's been spectacular," Jonathan said.

If your recipe collection doesn't include a flawless shepherd's pie recipe, it definitely does now. *Spectacular*, come to think of it, is a fitting word.

FOODIE TRUCK'S SHEPHERD'S PIE

Makes 8 to 10 servings.

Gather it up

4 tablespoons canola oil

1 pound ground lamb

1 pound ground beef

2 tablespoons extra virgin olive oil

1 cup finely diced yellow onion

½ cup peeled and diced (¼ inch) carrots

¼ teaspoon red pepper flakes

1 tablespoon chopped garlic

1 teaspoon minced fresh rosemary

1 teaspoon fresh thyme leaves

1 teaspoon chopped fresh oregano

1 tablespoon all-purpose flour

2 ounces dry red wine

1 ½ cups chicken stock

¾ cup tomato sauce

¼ cup ketchup

1 teaspoon Worcestershire sauce

2 cups cooked Yukon Gold potatoes

6 tablespoons cold, unsalted butter, cut into small pieces

1 cup heavy cream, heated

Salt to taste

½ cup frozen English peas

Make it happen

Preheat the oven to 400.

Place a large, heavy-bottomed stock pot over medium heat. Add the oil, and once it begins to shimmer or bead up in the pan, add the ground lamb and beef. Using a rubber spatula or wooden spoon, break up the meat, constantly stirring until there are no large pieces. Brown the meat slowly, stirring occasionally until a fond develops on the bottom of the pan. Drain the cooked meat in a colander or strainer.

In the same pot used to cook the meat, add the olive oil, onion, carrots, and pepper flakes to the pan, and cook over low heat. Cook until the vegetables are translucent and the carrots are tender. Add the garlic, rosemary, thyme, and oregano and continue to cook on low heat for 3 minutes.

Sift the flour over the pot and stir until well incorporated. Turn up the heat and quickly add the wine, constantly stirring and scraping the bottom of the pan to incorporate the caramelized bits stuck to the pan. Add the stock, tomato sauce, ketchup, Worcestershire sauce, and the reserved meat. Mix to combine. Once the mixture comes to a boil, reduce the heat to low.

Using a stand mixer with the paddle attachment, add the potatoes to the mixer bowl and mix on low. Add the butter a few pieces at a time, until melted and well incorporated. Pour the heated cream into the potato mixture and continue mixing until fully combined. Season with salt to taste.

To assemble the pie: Turn the heat off the meat filling, add the peas, and salt to taste. The filling should be wet but not soupy. Pour the meat into a 7 × 11-inch casserole dish and top with the potatoes, making sure to cover the meat mixture completely to prevent it from boiling over. Bake for 30 minutes or until the top of the potatoes begins to brown.

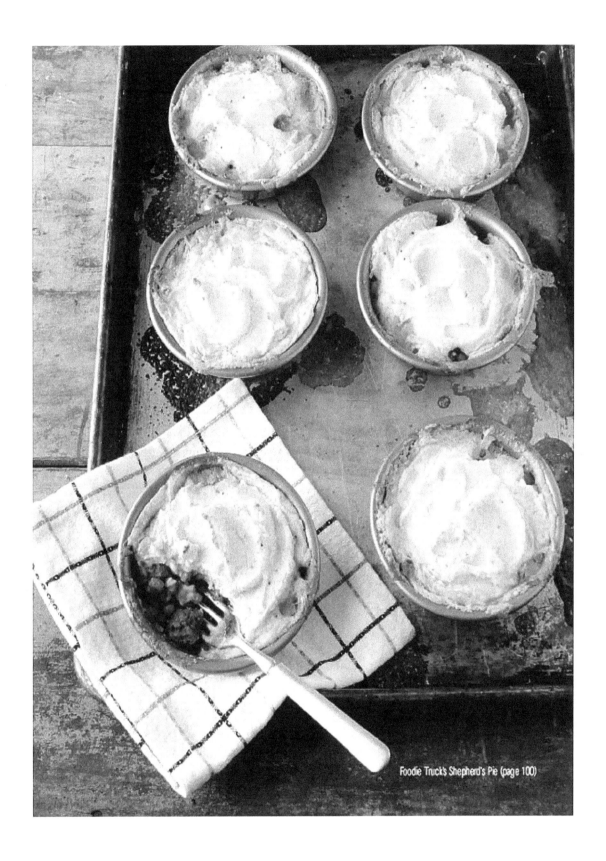

Foodie Truck's Shepherd's Pie (page 100)

DULCE TRUCK

SUMMERVILLE/CHARLESTON

Concept: Decadent desserts

dulcetruck.com

 facebook.com/DulceTruck

 Twitter: @DulceTruck

I don't know about you, but going to the beach and eating dessert are pretty much two of my favorite ways to spend time. It had never occurred to me how remarkable it might be to combine the two until I heard about Charleston's pretty pink Dulce Truck. Owned by Ericka Kalinowski and her husband, Michael, Dulce Truck dishes up high-end treats and infused sweet teas to locals and indulgent tourists all over the Holy City.

What should I order?

Vanilla bean cheesecake topped with caramel and bacon. You'll never forget it.

Ericka and Michael are both trained pastry chefs, and after watching new food trucks pop up all over Charleston, they realized they had something unique to offer on the street food scene. So they pooled their baking expertise; drafted up a menu of cookies, bars, cakes, Danishes, muffins, and scones; painted their truck pink; and hit the road. Any day at Dulce Truck might find a chalkboard boasting everything from crème brûlée and peanut butter bars, to chocolate ganache cake and bacon scones with blue cheese glaze. To round things out, they decided to develop a selection of flavor-infused sweet teas, brewed daily with local Charleston Tea Plantation tea, in flavors such as blueberry-basil, lemon-lavender, and green tea horchata.

And because every home cook needs a perfect chocolate cake recipe, Ericka shared hers, along with her technique for a simple peach iced tea.

DOUBLE-LAYER CHOCOLATE CAKE

Makes 12 to 16 slices.

Gather it up

2 cups sugar

1 cup butter, softened

1 teaspoon vanilla

2 eggs

2 ½ cups cake flour

1 cup cocoa powder

2 teaspoons baking soda

½ teaspoon salt

1 (12-ounce) bottle porter*

¾ cup milk

Chocolate Buttercream Icing (recipe follows)

Make it happen

Preheat the oven to 350 degrees and grease two 9-inch cake pans.

In a large bowl cream the sugar and butter until light and fluffy. Add the eggs and vanilla and mix just until they have combined with the butter and sugar. In a medium bowl stir together the cake flour, cocoa powder, baking soda, and salt. Add half of the flour mixture to the egg and butter mixture, along with the porter and milk. Mix for about 30 seconds and then add the remainder of the flour mixture. Mix on medium speed for about 1 minute or until well combined, scraping down the sides of the bowl thoroughly to incorporate well. Pour the batter into the prepared cake pans and bake for 30 to 40 minutes. Cool thoroughly before icing with Chocolate Buttercream Icing.

* Ericka likes locally produced Palmetto Brewery Espresso Porter, a particularly hoppy, dark beer.

CHOCOLATE BUTTERCREAM ICING

Makes about 3 ½ cups.

Gather it up

½ cup chocolate chips

3 cups powdered sugar, sifted

1 cup butter, softened

½ cup vegetable shortening

1 teaspoon vanilla extract

2 tablespoons milk or heavy cream

Make it happen

Place the chocolate in a microwavable bowl and heat in the microwave for two 15-second intervals, mixing well in between. If some of the chips are still whole, return the bowl to the microwave for 7 to 10 seconds at a time until it's all melted.

In a stand mixer fitted with a paddle attachment, combine the powdered sugar, butter, shortening, vanilla, and milk or cream. Start out on slow speed, and once all ingredients have been incorporated, turn the speed up to medium high and continue for about 3 minutes.

Turn the speed down to low and slowly pour in the melted chocolate. Once it's all in, increase the speed to high and mix for another 3 minutes or until light and fluffy. Be sure to scrape the bottom of the bowl once or twice to thoroughly incorporate all the ingredients.

PEACH SPICE SWEET TEA

Makes 1 gallon.

Gather it up

3 fresh South Carolina peaches (use the freshest you can find)

1 gallon water, divided

½ cup black tea leaves

3 crushed cardamom pods

1 cinnamon stick

Sugar to taste

Mint sprigs, for garnish

Make it happen

Cut the peaches into chunks and place in a blender with 2 cups of the water and blend until semi-smooth. Pour into a large nonreactive pot with the remaining water, tea leaves, cardamom pods, and cinnamon stick. Bring to a boil and then shut off. Let it sit in the pot for 10 minutes to infuse the flavors. Strain, cool, and sweeten with sugar to desired taste. Serve on ice with a sprig of mint.

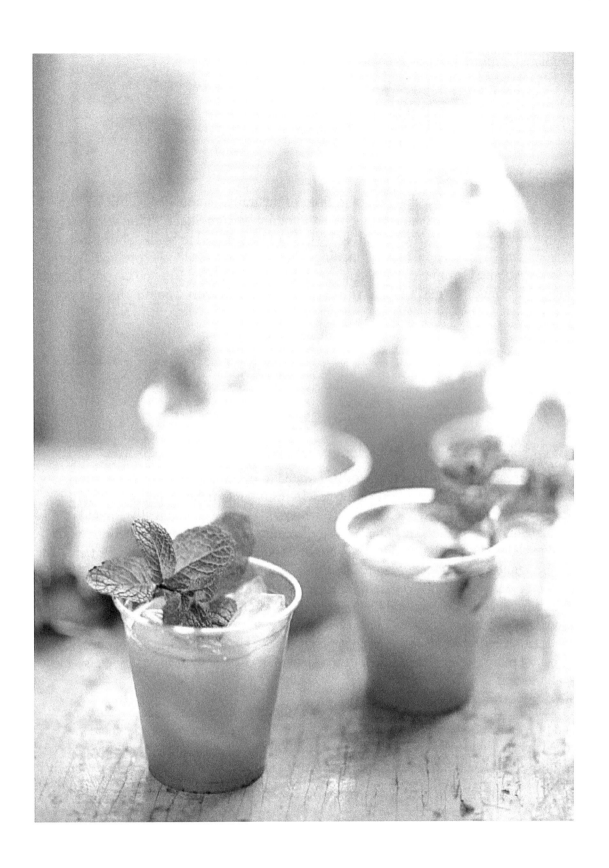

CAST IRON GRILL

CHARLESTON

Concept: Southern comfort, the cast-iron way

castiron-foodtruck.com

 facebook.com/CastironFoodTruck

 Twitter: @CastironTruck

The day I visited Cast Iron Grill, a chalkboard in front of the trailer announced, "Official Rule Change . . . Dessert is now the first course . . . Bread Pudding w/Rum Sauce." I immediately realized this was one (and perhaps the only) rule I wouldn't be tempted to break. Spurred on by this thrilling command, I ordered that bread pudding, along with the Mad Cap Portobello Mushroom Sandwich, the Carolina BBQ, and an order of collard greens. But you can bet I dug into that boozy bread pudding first! Cast Iron Grill owner Victor Colbert wouldn't have it any other way.

What should I order?

Can't go wrong with the Bob Marley Jerk Chicken Sandwich!

As a culinary student in the midnineties, Victor had hoped to eventually become an executive chef. After a handful of career detours, including one in restaurant kitchen management and another in mobile communications, Victor realized he wasn't doing what he really wanted to do. He longed to have his hands in the kitchen every day, creating recipes and experimenting with new ideas. It dawned on him that a food truck could be his ticket back into the culinary field. The versatility of the venue and the freedom to reshape his menu whenever he wanted was an exciting prospect. He knew he didn't want to be boxed in by a specific cuisine, and it occurred to him that the cast-iron concept gave him lots of breathing room. "You can cook everything in cast iron—cornbread, jerk chicken, pineapple upside-down cake, vegetables," Victor told me. "I also knew I wanted barbecue to be one aspect of the operation too, but I realized that most people these days are a lot more health conscious. Cast iron allows me to do all of those things, so the name just made sense."

Victor was more than happy to hand over the recipe for that Mad Cap Portobello Mushroom Sandwich, and I couldn't be happier to have it for my own recipe collection. Somewhere between the savory marinade and the cast-iron char, this sandwich winds up with all the meaty flavor of a burger. It's cast-iron magic!

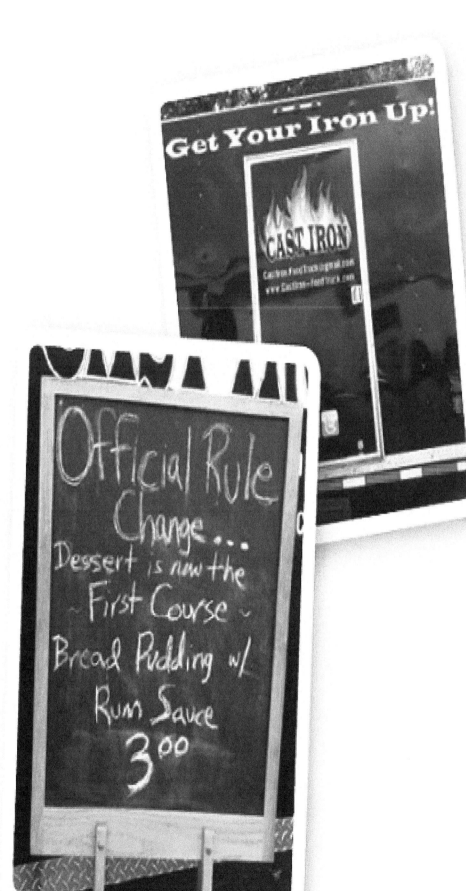

MAD CAP PORTOBELLO MUSHROOM SANDWICH

Makes 6 sandwiches.

Gather it up

Vegetable oil

6 Marinated Portobello Mushrooms (recipe follows)

6 ciabatta rolls

3 tablespoons butter, softened

1 ½ cups pesto mayonnaise (1 cup mayonnaise and ½ cup prepared pesto)

1 (12-ounce) package buffalo mozzarella cheese, sliced

1 ½ cups roasted red bell peppers, julienned

1 ½ cups fried onion straws

1 ½ cups mesclun salad mix

½ cup balsamic vinegar

Make it happen

Place a cast-iron grill pan over medium-high heat and grease with oil. Add the mushrooms to the pan and cook for 3 minutes on each side to heat throughout. Slice the ciabatta, spread the top part with butter, and toast. Spread the pesto on the bottom half of the rolls. Place the mozzarella and roasted red peppers on the gill side of the hot mushrooms until the cheese is slightly melted. Place the mushrooms on the bottom half of the rolls and top with the fried onion straws. Serve with mesclun salad and drizzle with balsamic vinegar.

MARINATED PORTOBELLO MUSHROOMS

Makes 6 portobello mushrooms caps.

Gather it up

½ cup balsamic vinegar

½ cup white wine

4 tablespoons dark soy sauce

2 tablespoons sesame oil

3 garlic cloves, finely minced

6 portobello caps, 5 inches in diameter

Make it happen

Combine the vinegar, white wine, soy sauce, sesame oil, and garlic in a stainless steel bowl, and whisk for 2 to 3 minutes. Add the portobello mushrooms to the marinade, gill side down (the gills are the thin brown layers on the underside of the mushroom). Marinate at least 2 hours, turning twice. Move the mushrooms to a clean container for storage and reserve the marinade for basting.

GEORGIA

King of Pops

Tangerine Basil Pops

Banana Puddin' Pops

Ibiza Bites

Fresh from the Patch Watermelon Gazpacho with Spiced Summer Pop

Sola Crispy Fried Green Tomatoes Stuffed with Goat Cheese and Spiked with Chipotle Aioli

Happy Belly Curbside Kitchen

Kale Waldorf Salad

Kippered Salmon

Farm Cart

Farm Cart Burger with Green Tomato Marmalade and Roasted Poblano Cheese

The Pickle

Yellow Heirloom Tomato Gazpacho with Crab

Southwestern Chicken Rollups

Honeysuckle Gelato

Honeydew Mint Sorbet

Crème Fraîche Gelato

Invert Sugar

Grace's Goodness

Georgia Apple Salad with Candied Pecans and Fennel

KING OF POPS

ATLANTA (ALSO RICHMOND, VIRGINIA, AND CHARLESTON, SOUTH CAROLINA)

Concept: All-natural handmade paletas

kingofpops.net

 facebook.com/kingofpops

 Twitter: @theKingofPops

It's almost too obvious to say, but I'm going for it anyway. There is simply nothing better than an icy cold paleta when you're standing in the surging heat of a Southern summer. Nothing. Originating in South America, these ice pops are similar to a good old Popsicle, but a little more interesting—made of fruits, herbs, and spices, and in the case of King of Pops, lots of other flavors too. There's Strawberry Peppercorn and Coconut with Toasted Almond, Chocolate Sea Salt and Apple Spinach Ginger, Coffee & Donuts and Grapefruit IPA. And that's only the beginning.

What should I order?

Chocolate Sea Salt or Blackberry Ginger Lemonade.

Steven Carse, who hatched the idea for King of Pops with his brothers, has concocted hundreds of paleta recipes since 2009. Understandably, not every flavor is available all the time, and frustratingly, it would be nearly impossible to ever taste them all. My trip, bless it, afforded me the chance to sample a couple of Steven's recipes—Lemon Basil and Watermelon Cucumber Lime—from King of Pops' cute little pushcarts in Richmond and Atlanta respectively. Both paletas had me dreading the end—those last few juicy bites from the wooden stick. It's hard to prepare for the end of a paleta.

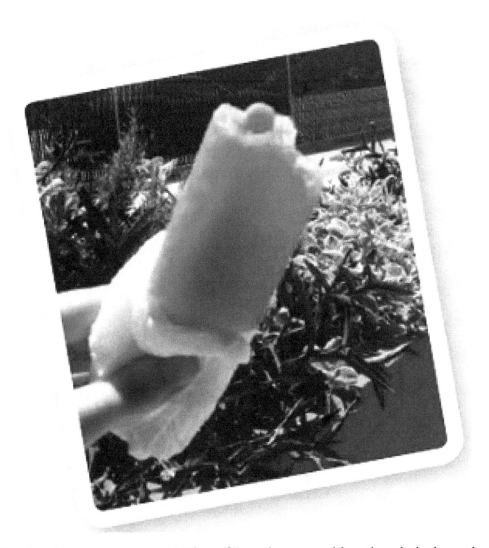

But here's some great news! King of Pops has several locations in its home base of Atlanta, as well as ones in Athens, Georgia; Richmond, Virginia; and Charleston, South Carolina. The first order of business, though, is for you to head to kingofpops.net and peruse the menu. It's a delight just to read it! Once your taste buds are all hot and bothered, scoot yourself into the kitchen and whip up your own paletas!

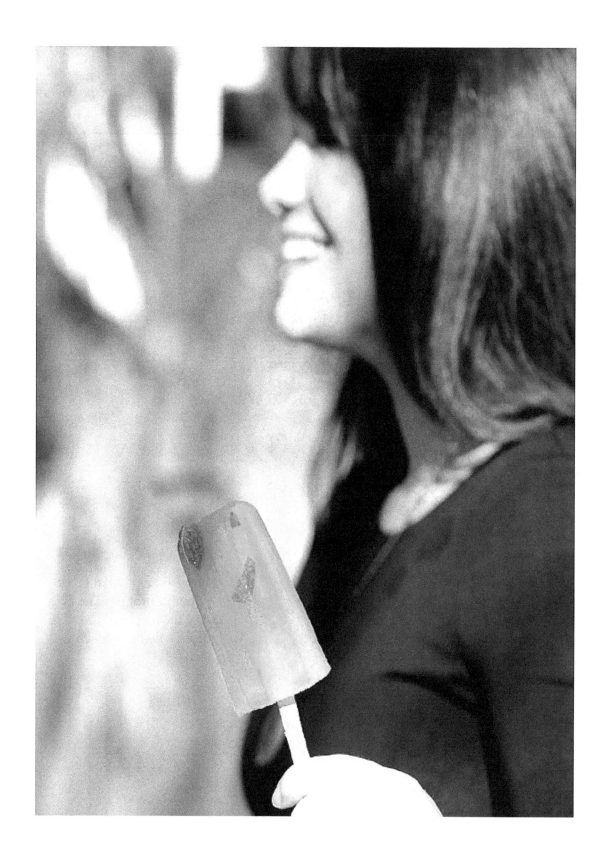

TANGERINE BASIL POPS

Makes 8 to 12 pops.

Gather it up

2 ¼ cups water

1 cup chopped fresh sweet basil

½ cup organic evaporated cane juice

Pinch of sea salt

3 cups fresh tangerine juice

⅛ cup fresh lemon juice

Make it happen

Pour the water into a large pot and add the chopped basil. Bring to a boil over high heat. Reduce to low heat and simmer, stirring occasionally for 30 minutes. Remove from the heat. Stir in the cane juice and sea salt and let steep with the basil for 12 hours at room temperature (if left out over 12 hours put it in the refrigerator). Strain through a fine-mesh sieve twice. Add the tangerine and lemon juice and stir to combine. Pour into molds and add a garnish of chopped basil to the top before putting sticks in. Freeze for 8 hours.

BANANA PUDDIN' POPS

Makes 16 (3-ounce) pops.

Gather it up

1 quart whole milk

½ cup heavy cream

1 vanilla bean, seeds scraped (keep seeds and pod)

1 ½ cups organic evaporated cane juice

8 ripe bananas, divided

32 bite-size vanilla wafers

Make it happen

In a saucepan over low heat mix the milk, cream, and vanilla (both scraped seeds and pod), and cane juice until warmed through. Remove from heat and let cool. Remove the vanilla pod.

Pour the liquid into a blender. Add 4 bananas and blend the mixture until smooth. Slice the 4 remaining bananas into 1-inch-thick pieces. Place two slices of banana and two vanilla wafers into each Popsicle mold. Then pour the milk mixture into the mold. Place one Popsicle stick in each mold, submerging it halfway. Freeze for at least 8 hours.

* The Carses recommend Nilla Wafers.

IBIZA BITES

ATLANTA

Concept: SoLa cuisine (deep South meets South America!)

iIbizabites.com

 facebook.com/ibizabites

 Twitter: @IbizaBites

If you live in the South, or even if you've spent any time eating in the South between June and September, you know what summer tastes like. It's corn and peaches, watermelon and tomatoes, with plenty of leafy goodness from the garden and something savory from the grill—maybe some heat from a homegrown chile too. At Ibiza Bites, Raf and Jamie Morales serve the sort of food I get giddy over—lots of produce, lots of herbs, tender meats, and flourishes of ethnic interest scattered throughout. I discovered their truck in Atlanta's hip Virginia Highlands neighborhood where an impromptu food truck park assembles on Thursday nights (for much of the year, anyway). The little parking lot was packed with sundresses and seersucker shorts and sandaled feet—dozens of people queuing up at the different trucks. Ibiza Bites boasted the longest line—a line I stood in three separate times after each order impressed me more than the last. I began with the grilled Georgia Peach Caprese Salad—all sweet and veggie fresh, with honey vinaigrette, creamy little balls of baby mozzarella and heirloom cherry tomatoes on a layer of arugula and basil. I followed it up with an order of Raf and Jamie's Lobster Mac & Cheese, and chased it all down with a fresh-squeezed mojito lemonade, so bright and cold.

What should I order?

SoLa A La Plancha: skirt steak with béarnaise butter, smashed acorn and butternut squashes with grilled green onion.

While I can't imagine any time of year when this menu wouldn't appeal to me, Ibiza Bites serves summer food at its best. Of course, the Moraleses adapt their menu with the changing seasons, but I was truly bowled over by how beautifully their menu captured the moment. Jamie happily shared a few beautiful examples of that flavor here. After you've sampled these dishes, check out the Ibiza Bites menu for yourself, and see if you're not inspired to try your hand at a few new seasonal delights.

IBIZA BITES
SPECIALS
• • • • • •

Sugar Cane Grilled Salmon
Pacific NW Salmon topped with a
Brown Sugar Lime glaze and served
with Sugar Snap Pea Beans Farmers Salad
with Sherry Vinaigrette **$12**

New Mexican Rubbed
Pork Tenderloin w/
B~~SOLD OUT~~ ~~auce~~
atop smashed Sweet potatoes
& a dried olive Rice

$10

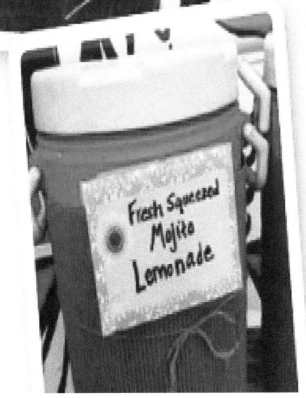

Fresh Squeezed
Mojito
Lemonade

FRESH FROM THE PATCH WATERMELON GAZPACHO WITH SPICED SUMMER POP

Makes 4 servings.

Gather it up

1 ½ cups Bloody Mary mix

½ serrano chile

2 cups cubed fresh red and yellow watermelon, divided

1 teaspoon sherry vinegar

¼ cup extra virgin olive oil

2 tablespoons minced red onion

½ cucumber, seeded and minced

1 tablespoon chopped Italian parsley

2 tablespoons minced chives, plus more for garnish

Kosher salt and black pepper to taste

Spiced Summer Pop (recipe follows)

Fresh blackberries, for garnish

Make it happen

In a blender add the Bloody Mary mix, chile, and 1 cup of the watermelon. Pour in the sherry vinegar and olive oil and pulse to blend. Add the onion, cucumber, parsley, and chives, and season with salt and pepper. Puree until smooth. Pour into chilled bowls and garnish with a sprinkling of chives, remaining watermelon, the Spiced Summer Pop, and fresh blackberries.

SPICED SUMMER POP

Makes 4 pops.

Gather it up

8 ounces Bloody Mary mix

1 cup diced watermelon

Make it happen

The day before you plan to serve the gazpacho, combine the Bloody Mary mix with the diced watermelon and pour into 4-ounce Popsicle trays. Freeze until ready to serve.

SOLA CRISPY FRIED GREEN TOMATOES STUFFED WITH GOAT CHEESE AND SPIKED WITH CHIPOTLE AIOLI

Makes 4 to 6 servings.

Gather it up

3 medium firm green tomatoes

1 tablespoon salt, plus extra for sprinkling on the tomatoes

½ cup peanut or vegetable oil

½ cup goat cheese

1 egg

½ cup heavy cream

1 cup all-purpose flour

½ Panko bread crumbs

Chipotle Aioli (recipe follows)

Make it happen

Cut the unpeeled tomatoes into ½-inch slices. Sprinkle the slices with salt. Let the slices stand for 5 minutes.

Heat the peanut oil in a skillet on medium heat. Roll the goat cheese into cherry-size balls. Press the goat cheese balls on the tomato slices and spread evenly over tomato.

In a shallow bowl beat the egg and the heavy cream together. In another shallow bowl combine the flour and salt. Pour the bread crumbs into a third shallow bowl. Dip the tomato slices in the flour-salt mixture, then the cream-egg mixture, and finally in the bread crumbs. Carefully place half of the breaded tomato slices in the skillet and fry for 3 to 5 minutes on each side or until brown. Set the cooked tomatoes on a wire cooling rack to drain the excess oil. Repeat with the remaining breaded slices. Serve with a drizzle of Chipotle Aioli.

Raf says: "This may be served atop Southern stone ground Cheddar grits."

CHIPOTLE AIOLI

Makes 4 to 6 servings.

Gather it up

1 cup mayonnaise

2 chipotle chiles in adobo, minced

1 tablespoon fresh lime juice

1 teaspoon honey

1 teaspoon soy sauce

½ teaspoon sesame oil

Make it happen

In a medium bowl whisk together the mayonnaise, chiles, lime juice, honey, soy sauce, and sesame oil. Serve with fried green tomatoes and refrigerate any remaining aioli.

HAPPY BELLY CURBSIDE KITCHEN

ATLANTA/SMYRNA

Concept: Farm-to-street fresh

happybellytruck.com

 facebook.com/HappyBellyTruck

 Twitter: @happybellytruck

For me, one of the most exciting experiences of eating from a food truck is watching the owner's face as I take my first bite of whatever he or she has just handed me. There's an expectant expression there. It's the sort of sincere excitement you don't often see when eating out, and I love that. It's thrilling to know that the person serving your food gets such a huge kick out of seeing you make a "wow-this-is-incredible" face. Terry Hall gets to see those looks pretty frequently as the owner of Happy Belly Curbside Kitchen. He and his wife, Dawn, started the operation as an extension of their own food philosophy. When their daughter was born, they decided to only feed her fresh, natural foods. The snag in that plan was that foods falling into those categories weren't always so easy to find when they were on the go.

What should I order?

Prepare to enjoy the best burger of your life (The Georgian!), with a side of the Kale Waldorf Salad.

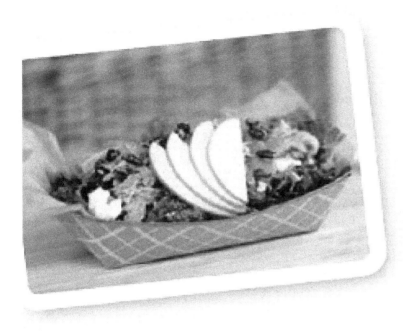

After realizing they couldn't possibly be the only family who felt that way, Terry and Dawn came up with their own solution to a problem they believed others had encountered. Happy Belly is their answer to the fast/healthy dilemma. Judging by their standing as one of Atlanta's most popular food trucks, Terry and Dawn obviously had the right answer. *SHAPE* magazine even named Happy Belly one of the ten healthiest food trucks in the country.

Now, before you go imagining a truck full of nothing but quinoa and kale (which Happy Belly serves in beautifully delicious treatments), guess again. The Halls work closely with local Georgia farmers and chefs to create in-season menus that feature perfectly herbed free-range chicken, short-rib brisket, and kippered salmon. The secret to healthy but delicious food, as we all know, lies in the preparation and the quality of the ingredients. Turns out, Happy Belly is the only food truck in the world to be sponsored by Big Green Egg, meaning they have one of the company's world-famous smokers built right into the truck. Fresh ingredients? Check! Flavor-infusing prep method? Yup! Even better, Happy Belly donates 5 percent of its profits to the Boys and Girls Clubs of Metro Atlanta.

Terry and Dawn have even bigger plans for Happy Belly . . . plans that may or may not involve a presence throughout the Southeast. Cross your fingers on that, and in the meantime, add Happy Belly to your must-eat list for Atlanta. And if you can't make it to Atlanta right away, just be glad that Terry was amazing enough to divulge one of Happy Belly's signature recipes—the illustrious Kale Waldorf Salad. If you think you don't like kale, this salad will change everything for you.

KALE WALDORF SALAD

Makes 4 servings.

Gather it up

1 Granny Smith apple, chopped

1 tablespoon honey

1 tablespoon Dijon mustard

3 tablespoons canola oil (more if needed)

1 tablespoon cider vinegar

⅛ teaspoon sea salt

4 cups packed finely chopped raw kale*

2 D'Anjou pears, chopped

½ cup blue cheese

½ cup roasted pecans

¼ cup plus 2 tablespoons raisins

Make it happen

To make the dressing: Place the apple, honey, mustard, oil, vinegar, and salt in a blender. Puree until well combined and slightly thick. Add water, if needed, to thin.

To prepare the salad: Place the kale in a large bowl. Pour the dressing over the kale, toss to combine, and let rest for 5 minutes to soften the kale. Add the pears, blue cheese, pecans, and raisins to the bowl and toss.

* *Happy Belly uses Scotch kale.*

Note: Can top salad with Kippered Salmon (recipe on page 130).

KIPPERED SALMON

Makes 6 servings.

Gather it up

1 (1 ½-to 2-pound) Atlantic salmon side, skin on

1 cup brown sugar

1 cup coarse kosher salt

Applewood chips

All-natural hardwood charcoal

Make it happen

Pat the salmon dry. Mix the brown sugar and salt and apply generously to salmon filet. Wrap with plastic wrap and refrigerate a minimum of 24 hours. Remove the salmon from the wrap and rinse thoroughly under cool water. Place the applewood chips in a shallow container and cover with water. Soak for at least 30 minutes.

Bring a grill to 220 to 225 degrees. Add the wet applewood chips to the grill. Put the salmon over indirect heat and allow to cook for approximately 20 minutes. The internal temperature of the salmon should be no more than 115 degrees when pulled from the grill. Immediately put the salmon in the refrigerator so the fish does not continue to cook. Salmon should have a brilliant pink color with plenty of visible moisture. Pull the meat from the skin once cooled and serve atop kale salad.

FARM CART

ATHENS

Concept: Farm-fresh fare

farm255.com/farmcart

facebook.com/Farm255

Twitter: @Farm255

You might think of Farm Cart as an evangelist to the masses, spreading the good news of sustainable dining in an accessible way. As a spinoff of Athens's highly acclaimed Farm 255 restaurant, Farm Cart began as a way to broaden access to the experience of farm-to-table dining. "Sustainable food doesn't have to be elitist," Olivia Sargeant of Farm 255 told me. "We wanted to offer up the Farm 255 ethos in a beautiful and fun way."

What should I order?

The Farm Cart Burger is hard to pass up, but if you're not feeling especially carnivorous, try the Southern Vegetable Banh Mi, made with marinated carrots, onions, and cucumbers with cilantro and smoked egg salad.

The Farm 255 family of eateries sources its menus seasonally and sustainably, thanks to its own farm and livestock operation. Anything they don't happen to grow or raise themselves, they get from local organic farmers. Farm Cart began as a fun way for Farm 255 to serve lunch on its patio, offering their signature flavors in an easier format and at a lower price point. In 2012, Farm Cart struck out from its home at the restaurant and is now a regular at the Athens Farmers

Market, local events, and private shindigs. The rustic-chic Farm Cart has even been known to surface in Atlanta for events with the city's Street Food Coalition.

"It's party whimsy, part kitsch, part function," Olivia said. "Yes, we're a fine-dining establishment, but we can do so much more than that."

Until you can get to Athens, treat yourself to this replica of the Farm Cart Burger at home. And if you really want to see what the fuss is all about, be sure to use organic grass-fed beef!

FARM CART BURGER WITH GREEN TOMATO MARMALADE AND ROASTED POBLANO CHEESE

Makes 4 burgers.

Gather it up

1 ¾ pounds organic beef

Salt and black pepper to taste

4 good-quality sandwich buns

Poblano Cheese (recipe follows)

Green Tomato Marmalade (recipe follows)

Make it happen

Divide the beef into four 6-ounce patties and season liberally with salt and pepper. Preheat the grill or a grill pan over medium-high heat. Oil the grates or grease the grill pan. Cook the burgers for 3 minutes on each side for medium-rare. (Farm Cart suggests medium-rare.)

Bring it all together

Toast the buns and top each burger patty with a scoop of Poblano Cheese. Add the Green Tomato Marmalade to the bottom half of the bun, then add the cheese-topped burger.

POBLANO CHEESE

Makes 2 ⅔ cups.

Gather it up

2 poblano peppers

3 ounces cream cheese, softened

2 cups sharp white Cheddar cheese, shredded

½ cup mayonnaise*

1 tablespoon black pepper

Salt to taste

Make it happen

Roast the poblanos over an open flame until charred on all sides, then place in a bowl and cover with plastic wrap. Once the peppers are cool enough to handle, peel and dice them.

Combine the peppers, cream cheese and Cheddar, mayonnaise, pepper, and salt. Mix until well combined. Serve immediately on the burgers, or cover and refrigerate.

* Duke's brand if available.

GREEN TOMATO MARMALADE

Makes 1 pint.

Gather it up

1 pound green tomatoes, diced

Zest and juice of 1 orange

2 teaspoons fresh lemon juice

½ cup sugar

Pinch of salt

Make it happen

Combine the tomatoes, orange zest and juice, lemon juice, sugar, and salt in a bowl, cover, and let sit overnight.

In a medium saucepan bring the mixture to a boil over medium-high heat, turn the heat down to a simmer, and reduce until 1 cup remains (about 1 hour). Store refrigerated, in an airtight container.

Olivia says: "At Farm 255, we use grass-fed, hormone-and antibiotic-free beef raised on the Georgia pastures of the farmers in our meat cooperative, Moonshine Meats. The complex flavor profile of grass-fed beef is what makes our burgers great, and the only complement they need is a good bit of salt."

THE PICKLE

ATLANTA

Concept: South of the border meets the bayou

thepickleatl.com/pickle

facebook.com/pages/The-Pickle

 Twitter: @ThePickleAtl

Within every street food scene, there are those food trucks with reputations that precede them. Their loyal customers stalk them on Twitter. People show up at events they wouldn't ordinarily attend just so they can get a fix. The online reviews for these places soar into 5-star territory with lavish superlatives. In Atlanta, The Pickle is one of those (if not THE) trucks. Andy Grimes, the proud owner, is hard to miss when he shows up somewhere in The Pickle itself—his green 1975 GMC Palm Beach RV. When he's not selling out at lunch crowds, festivals, and weekend events, Andy keeps the hard-charging athletes of Atlanta's massive Ultimate Frisbee scene fueled up with his beer-battered cod tacos, Cajun chicken eggrolls, crab cake sandwiches, and nearly legendary crawfish etouffee. The Pickle is widely thought to be Atlanta's first gourmet food truck, having first hit the streets nearly a decade ago.

What should I order?

Ask for the Cajun Chicken and Tasso Ham Eggrolls, and join the legions of fans who are devoted to them.

After a long career at several big-name restaurants and in corporate catering, Andy lost his job in the post-9/11 downturn. "So I invented a new job," he said. "I was on the food service committee at my church, and in 2002, they were looking to upgrade what they were already doing, so I was able to sort of establish a catering company (Ultimate Catering) that kind of grew organically from there."

And from that, The Pickle emerged. Andy laughed, recalling his first event in the big green motorhome. "It was a Kanye West show with twenty-five thousand people," he said. "We were slammin' the food out, definitely trial by fire."

Try your hand at a couple of Andy's favorite recipes. These are two he once shared with a cooking class he taught. But be warned, Andy said the gazpacho's "not even worth making" unless you use fresh, ripe tomatoes!

YELLOW HEIRLOOM TOMATO GAZPACHO WITH CRAB

Makes 6 to 8 servings.

Gather it up

1 large red onion, chopped

2 red bell peppers, chopped

1 cucumber, peeled, seeded, and chopped

6 medium ripe yellow heirloom tomatoes, peeled and seeded

1 ½ teaspoons chopped garlic

1 ½ teaspoons kosher salt

½ teaspoon black pepper

¼ teaspoon cayenne pepper

1 tablespoon sherry wine vinegar

6 tablespoons extra virgin olive oil

1 tablespoon fresh lemon juice

½ tablespoon honey

1 cup cubed day-old bread, crust removed

1 sprig thyme

1 pound jumbo lump crabmeat*

Make it happen

In a large bowl mix the onion, red peppers, cucumber, tomatoes, garlic, salt, black and cayenne pepper, vinegar, oil, lemon juice, honey, bread, and thyme and refrigerate overnight. Remove the thyme sprig and puree the mixture in a blender. Adjust the seasoning as needed. Serve in chilled bowls and garnish each serving with crab meat.

* The Pickle uses blue crab, but feel free to use the best-quality crab you can find in your area.

Andy says: "It's best to roughly chop the vegetables and allow them to meld overnight to develop the flavors, but you can refrigerate for several hours in a pinch."

SOUTHWESTERN CHICKEN ROLLUPS

Makes 4 rollups.

Gather it up

1 (8-ounce) package cream cheese, softened

1 tablespoon fresh lime juice

¼ cup chopped fresh cilantro

½ teaspoon chopped garlic

1 teaspoon kosher salt

½ teaspoon black pepper

4 (10-inch) flour tortillas

1 (12-ounce) chicken breast, grilled and chopped

6 poblano peppers, roasted, peeled, and seeded

2 cups romaine lettuce, sliced thin

Make it happen

Mix the cream cheese, lime juice, cilantro, garlic, salt, and pepper together in a mixer or food processor. Place the tortillas on the countertop and spread the top two-thirds of each tortilla with ¼ cup of cilantro cream cheese. Starting at the bottom of each tortilla, add 3 ounces of chicken, 1 ½ poblanos cut into strips, and ½ cup of lettuce, leaving the top quarter of the tortilla without any ingredients except the cilantro cream cheese. Roll up the tortilla, working from the center to the outside to get a tight roll, and seal the tortilla with the cream cheese. Slice the rollup on the bias into thirds for sandwich portions or into 1-inch bias slices for appetizers.

HONEYSUCKLE GELATO

ATLANTA

Concept: Italian ice cream

honeysucklegelato.com

 facebook.com/pages/Honeysuckle-Gelato

Twitter: @honeysuckleatl

Everything about Honeysuckle Gelato is a delight—the imaginative flavors, the fun inky script on the side of the blue truck, and most especially, the story of the three people who run it.

What should I order?

Hard to go wrong with Honeysuckle's celebrated Sea-Salted Caramel flavor, but don't overlook the Honey Fig.

Jackson Smith, Wes Jones, and Khatera Ballard started Honeysuckle Gelato in 2011, merging three wildly different backgrounds into one very successful venture. Wes and Jackson are childhood pals who grew up together in Atlanta's Chastain Park neighborhood. After college, Wes headed to New Orleans for a stint with Teach for America (during Hurricane Katrina, no less), followed by a foray into commercial real estate in Atlanta. Meanwhile, Jackson did a good bit of globe-trotting, eventually landing in New York City, where he found himself immersed in the world of handcrafted gelato at Il Laboratorio del Gelato, under the guidance of gelato icon Jon Snyder.

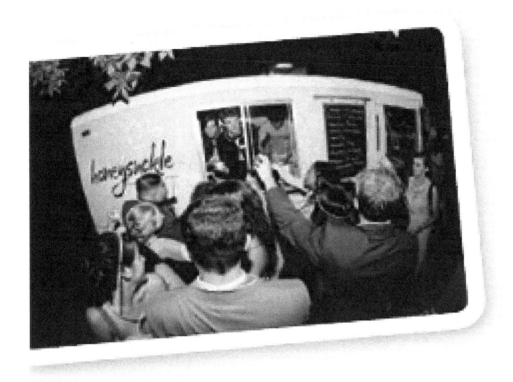

It wasn't long before Jackson began combining his newfound skill with the flavor profiles of his native palate. During visits home to Atlanta, Jackson started tinkering around with gelato and sorbet flavors reminiscent of classic Southern desserts, landing him rave reviews from friends and a solid demand for more. So he obliged, reconnecting with his old friend Wes over the idea of bringing artisan gelato home to Georgia.

Khatera, another of Jackson's friends, hopped on board with the idea, and Honeysuckle Gelato was born. Just two years later Honeysuckle Gelato's Southern-inspired desserts can be found in Atlanta's best restaurants, specialty grocery stores, and wherever their lovely blue truck happens to make an appearance. With flavors like Bourbon Pecan, Lunar Pastry (an homage to that famous Southern snack cake), and Ginger Molasses, there's a flavor for everyone.

Now you can try your hand at the gelato craft, thanks to these two great recipes Jackson put together, along with a mini lesson and equipment recommendations. Diverti, y'all!

Jackson says: "As far as machines go, I use the Delonghi gm6000, which has a self-contained cooling unit and is a little bit pricier. If you're thinking of making gelato or ice cream a serious hobby, I would highly recommend it. If you're just looking to whip up some fresh frozen treats for the family, Cuisinart has a few models for around fifty bucks that are more than capable."

HONEYDEW MINT SORBET

Makes 1 ½ pints.

Gather it up

24 ounces honeydew melon, cut into chunks (roughly half of a large melon)

½ cup invert sugar (recipe on page 145)

8 to 10 mint leaves

Make it happen

Place the chunks of the melon, invert sugar, and mint leaves in a blender and puree. Blend on high for about a minute or until completely smooth. Pour the mixture into the bowl of your ice-cream maker and process according to manufacturer's directions.

Note: This is an easy and refreshing sorbet to create. It can be enjoyed on a hot summer day to cleanse one's palate between courses, or even incorporated into savory dishes.

CRÈME FRAÎCHE GELATO

Makes 2 pints.

Gather it up

16 ounces whole milk

4 ounces heavy cream

8 ounces crème fraîche

4 ounces invert sugar (recipe on page 145)

Make it happen

Whisk the milk, cream, crème fraîche, and invert sugar in a large bowl until fully incorporated. Pour the mixture into the bowl of your ice-cream maker and process according to manufacturer's directions. It's possible to over-churn this recipe, so take it out a little early before it can truly solidify.

Jackson says: "This is one of my favorite batches to make because its rich dairy flavor pairs so well with jams. I prefer to serve it with a spoonful of fig preserves, but I would implore you to try it with as many fruits as you can."

INVERT SUGAR

Makes 4 cups and 6 tablespoons.

Gather it up

4 cups plus 6 tablespoons extra-fine granulated sugar

2 cups water

¼ teaspoon cream of tartar or citric acid

Make it happen

If you have an induction cooktop or an electric stove, these options are preferable to a gas stove. In a nonreactive saucepan over medium-high heat stir the sugar, water, and cream of tartar (or citric acid) until it begins to boil. Do not stir the mixture.

Once the mixture begins to boil, reduce the heat to medium and wash away any sugar crystals stuck to the side of the pan with a pastry brush dipped in water. Any additional water added to the pan from this process has no effect on the final outcome.

Boil the mixture to 236 degrees F (114 degrees C). Remove from the heat and cover the pan. Let cool at room temperature. Store in the refrigerator. Invert sugar will last at least 6 months.

GRACE'S GOODNESS

ATLANTA

Concept: Farm-fresh "fast food"

gracesgoodness.com

facebook.com/pages/Graces-Goodness

Twitter: @GracesGoodness

Brittany Grace Shiver spends a lot of time thinking about food. How it's grown. How it's prepared. How it's eaten. And while some of us may grab the organic strawberries when they're on sale, Brittany is completely devoted to the idea that what you eat shapes the way you live.

What should I order?

You've gotta go with the Mama's Pimento Cheese, a creamy blend of organic mayo, organic roasted red peppers, Tillamook sharp Cheddar cheese, crème fraîche, and freshly ground black pepper.

Her little food cart, Grace's Goodness, partners with local farmers and artisans to serve up portable and healthy options to one of the South's busiest cities. One Mason jar at a time, Brittany is making it easier for her community to eat the types of meals that will keep them nourished and healthy.

Grace's Goodness is the clean-food alternative to the local convenience store or deep-fried drive-thru. It's the sort of place that replaces potato chips and sodas with little jars of black-eyed pea hummus and icy watermelon aqua fresca. The jars are Brittany's way of making it easy (and portable) for you to eat as healthfully as possible, even when your schedule may prevent you from what she calls "intentional eating"—purposely eating the right foods when you're genuinely hungry.

"There's something for everyone," she promised. "You can grab a quick lunch, or you can grab provisions to help you make it through the rest of your school or work week healthfully."

Brittany understands that the bounty from local farmers and health food markets isn't always accessible to the average person. That's why she's trying to bridge the gap between busy schedules and smart food choices. Best of all? You can bring your Mason jar back the next time you visit Grace's Goodness, and Brittany'll fill 'er up with your favorites.

To give you an idea of the garden-fresh flavors you'll find at Grace's Goodness, she handed over one of her favorite salad recipes.

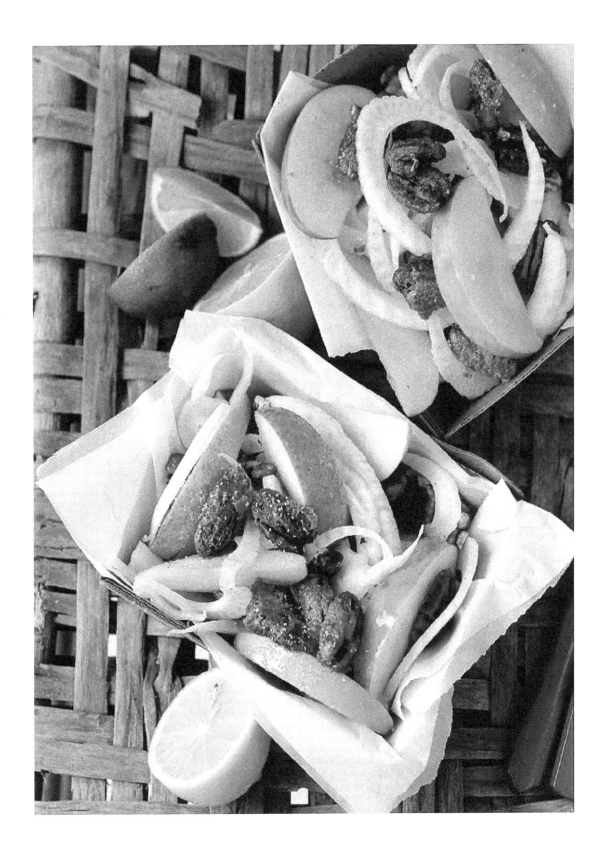

GEORGIA APPLE SALAD WITH CANDIED PECANS AND FENNEL

Makes 12 servings.

Gather it up

Juice of 1 lime

Juice of 1 lemon

2 tablespoons extra virgin olive oil

Salt and black pepper to taste

5 to 6 apples of various textures and colors, sliced into ½-inch-thick slices, lengthwise

1 fennel bulb, finely sliced

2 cups Candied Pecans (recipe follows)

Make it happen

To make the dressing: Whisk the lime and lemon juice together in a small bowl. Slowly drizzle in the olive oil until the desired consistency is reached. Add the salt and pepper to taste.

To assemble the salad: Toss the apple slices in a little bit of the dressing. Place in a bowl and refrigerate. Do the same with the fennel pieces but leave separate. After at least 30 minutes, add the fennel to the apple and sprinkle the Candied Pecans on top. Add more citrus dressing if desired.

CANDIED PECANS

Makes 4 cups.

Gather it up

1 egg white

Sprinkle of fresh nutmeg, ground cloves, and cayenne pepper

¾ cup brown sugar

½ teaspoon ground ginger

¼ teaspoon salt

2 teaspoons vanilla extract

1 pound pecan halves

Make it happen

Preheat the oven to 325 degrees. Line a baking sheet with parchment paper. In a medium bowl combine the egg white, nutmeg, cloves, pepper, brown sugar, ground ginger, salt, and vanilla, and stir until fully incorporated. Add the pecans and stir gently until they are evenly coated. Place on the prepared baking sheet and bake for 30 minutes.

Brittany says: "Real vanilla extract never leaves a metallic aftertaste and will preserve the tasty quality of your treats!"

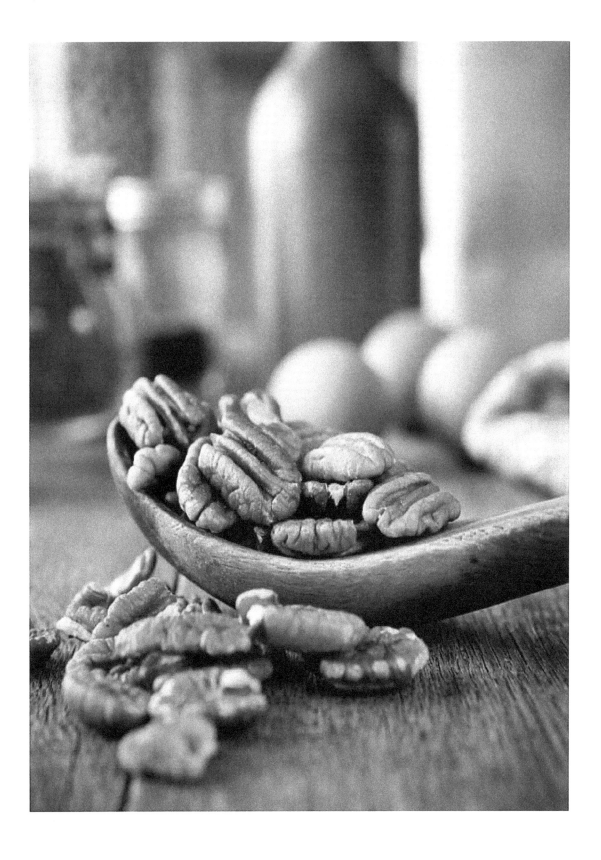

ALABAMA

Spoonfed Grill

THE SOUTHERN SOUL BOWL

Slow-Roasted Pork

Morita Salsa

Kick'n Collards

Lime-Thyme Sauce

Tomato Chutney

Roasted Sweet Potatoes

Fresh Off the Bun

Caramelized Pork

Sesame Noodle Salad

SPOONFED GRILL

BIRMINGHAM

Concept: Gourmet Southern fusion

spoonfedgrill.com

 facebook.com/sfgrill

Twitter: @SpoonFedGrill

Michael Brandon is a chef. He's not an astronaut. But in 2009, when he hit the streets of Birmingham in the Spoonfed Grill truck with partner and founder Jason Parkman, he said it felt like he'd just landed on the moon.

What should I order?

Order any main dish you like, but be sure your meal includes the roasted sweet potatoes and cilantro lime rice.

"People were like, 'What is this thing? Is it safe?'" Michael remembered, amused. "Then people started trying it out, and it all changed. They were like, 'Oh, that's awesome! What do you have today?'"

On any given day, the answer to that question can vary. Some days he's serving up his popular Cherry Steak Roll-Up, with seared petite tenderloin, blue cheese, and cherry preserves. Catch him another day, and the Latin Soul Bowl may be up for grabs with its fried Jack cheese grits, spinach, orange marinated chicken, and tomatillo salsa. While much of Spoonfed Grill's menu is consistently available, Michael is driven to keep things interesting.

Like so many other food truckers, Michael had spent his previous career in a windowless, stainless-steel restaurant kitchen. While he loved the work, he was feeling a bit boxed in and longed to be outside more, around other people. Partnering with Jason Parkman on the Spoonfed Grill venture fit the bill on both counts. Over the last several years, Michael has been an outspoken proponent for Birmingham's street food scene, advocating for ordinances that don't hinder the continued development of mobile dining.

When I asked Michael for a couple of recipes, he ignored me and promptly sent over a party instead. The Southern Soul Bowl, Michael said, is his "absolute favorite thing" he produces on the truck. "I want to share it with the world!" he told me.

This six-part recipe requires some planning, but Michael walks you through every step of the process. I suggest trying out this incredible creation the next time you invite a crowd over to watch the big game, but plan ahead! You'll need two days to pull everything together.

DAY 1

• Purchase all the ingredients.

• Make the Slow-Roasted Pork.

• Reserve the pork jus and pork fat.

• Assemble the Tomato Chutney or purchase fig preserves.

DAY 2

• Prep the ingredients for the Roasted Sweet Potatoes and make the Lime-Thyme Sauce.

• Cook the Kick'n Collards.

• Reheat the pork.

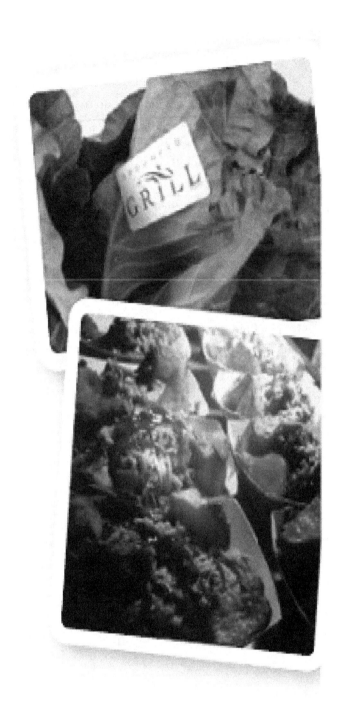

THE SOUTHERN SOUL BOWL

Makes 24 servings.

SLOW-ROASTED PORK

Makes 20 servings.

Gather it up

1 (7 to 11 pound) Boston butt/pork shoulder, bone-in

1 cup brown sugar

1 cup salt

½ cup garlic salt

½ cup dried oregano

¼ cup black pepper

¼ cup chili powder

Morita Salsa (recipe follows)

Make it happen

Preheat the oven to 400 degrees. Rinse the pork under cold water, place on a cutting board, and cut a 1-inch patchwork lattice approximately 1 inch deep into the fat/skin side of the pork. Place the pork in a pan as deep as the pork is tall and wide.

In a medium bowl combine the brown sugar, salt, garlic salt, oregano, pepper, and chili powder. Rub 1 ½ cups of the spice mixture over the pork and into the lattice cuts. Add 2 to 3 cups of water to the pan, coming 2 inches up the sides of the pork. Cover the pan with foil and roast for 2 hours. Remove the foil, lower the oven temperature to 350 degrees, and continue to roast for an additional 2 hours. Remove the pork from the oven when the bone can be easily pulled out. Pour off the braising liquid and refrigerate to separate the pork fat from the pork jus. Reserve the pork jus.

Pull the pork and mix with 1 quart of the Morita Salsa. The pork will soak up the juices and be ready to serve or hold for up to a week with no loss in flavor.

MORITA SALSA

Makes 1 ½ quarts.

Gather it up

5 cups tomatillos

6 to 8 medium morita peppers*

2 tablespoons minced garlic

1 tablespoon salt

¼ cup red wine vinegar

Make it happen

Remove the husks from the tomatillos and place in a pot. Next, remove the stem end of the morita peppers and place in a pot. Fill the pot with cool water to the top of the tomatillos and place on the stovetop. Bring to a simmer over high heat. Immediately turn off the heat and remove from the stove. Drain in a colander. Allow to cool for several minutes before proceeding. Place the tomatillos, morita peppers, garlic, salt, and vinegar in the bowl of a blender** and process on high speed for 90 seconds. After blending, use a funnel to slowly pour the salsa into plastic squeeze bottles or another sealable container.

Morita peppers are smoked, red-ripe jalapeño peppers, much like the chipotle pepper. The main difference is that moritas are smoked for less time, which leaves them softer and retains their slightly fruity flavor. They are very richly flavored.

**Be very careful to remove the clear plastic cap on the blender top and cover with a clean towel to allow the steam to escape while processing.*

KICK'N COLLARDS

Makes 2 cups.

Gather it up

3 bunches collard greens

2 cups pork fat (bacon grease or lard)

2 white onions, julienned

3 tablespoons crushed red pepper flakes

¾ cup chopped garlic

1 quart reserved pork jus

1 gallon water

2 cups cider vinegar, divided

1 (32-ounce) can diced tomatoes, or 4 cups chopped fresh tomatoes

Make it happen

Pulling the leaves from the stems of the collard greens is the first and most important step. When the leaves are pulled from the stems, stack them as neatly as possible and cut into ribbons, 1 to 2 inches thick. Then cut those ribbons into uniformly sized squares. After all the leaves are cut to size, wash the greens thoroughly in several batches, removing all dirt and grit.

Heat a large saucepot or Dutch oven over high heat. Add the pork fat. Once it has melted and heated, add the onions. Cook over high heat without adding color for 3 to 5 minutes. Add the crushed red pepper and cook for another minute before adding the garlic to cook for 2 more minutes. Add the pork jus and water and bring to a boil.

Begin adding the collard greens a few handfuls at a time. As they wilt, more can be added until all have begun cooking together. Add 1 cup of the vinegar and continue to cook over medium-low heat for 30 to 45 minutes. Allow the water to come to a boil and add the tomatoes and remaining 1 cup of vinegar (you can add less if you want to), and cook to desired doneness. We like them to have a little bite or chew, but definitely not soggy.

LIME-THYME SAUCE

Makes about 1 ½ cups.

Gather it up

1 cup fresh lime juice

½ cup extra virgin olive oil

½ tablespoon garlic salt

1 tablespoon fresh thyme, minced

Make it happen

Place the lime juice, olive oil, garlic salt, and thyme in the bowl of a blender and mix to combine. Transfer to a plastic squeeze bottle or sealed container and refrigerate.

TOMATO CHUTNEY

Makes 2 cups.

Gather it up

1 jar prepared tomato chutney*

1 tablespoon white vinegar

Make it happen

Add the tomato chutney to the bowl of a blender. Pour the vinegar into the chutney jar, replace the lid, shake, open, and pour the remaining contents into the blender bowl. Cover the blender bowl and puree on high speed for 30 seconds or until fully combined. Pour the contents into a clear plastic bottle or a sealable container and refrigerate.

* Spoonfed Grill uses Alecia's brand Tomato Chutney and Fig Jam interchangeably.

ROASTED SWEET POTATOES

Makes 12 servings.

Gather it up

5 or 6 sweet potatoes

2 tablespoons canola oil

2 teaspoons salt

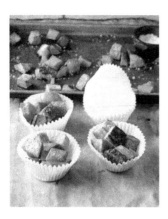

Make it happen

Preheat the oven to 400 degrees. Cut ⅛ inch off the ends of each sweet potato and peel. Cut each potato in half lengthwise, then cut each potato into pieces approximately the size of a Ping-Pong ball. Place these pieces into a large bowl and toss with the canola oil. Shake the salt over the potatoes and toss again to coat evenly. Spread the potatoes out on one or two sheet pans, and roast for 40 to 60 minutes until the largest pieces are easily pierced with a paring knife.

Bring it all together

Into a medium to large single serving bowl place a portion of the Kick'n Collards, then the Slow-Roasted Pork directly on top, surround with several of the Roasted Sweet Potato chunks, and top with the Tomato Chutney or fig preserves.

Michael says: "Enjoy this deliciousness, then go back for seconds."

FRESH OFF THE BUN

BIRMINGHAM

Concept: Vietnamese-Cajun

freshoffthebun.com

 facebook.com/Freshoffthebun

Twitter: @FreshofftheBun

Facts are facts. When you're born in Vietnam and raised in New Orleans, your standard for flavor might be a bit more demanding than that of the average palate (whatever that is). Luckily for Birmingham, Tosha Tran is sharing her flavorful culinary heritage with Fresh Off the Bun, a food truck known around Birmingham for creating meals that are as pleasing to taste buds as they are to waistlines. Having worked as a dialysis nurse, Tosha recognized the need for on-the-go food options that weren't grease-soaked, deep-fried, and teeming with sugar. "It's hard to find a fast meal that isn't full of fat and calories," Tosha said. "We don't have a lot of choices here, and I just kept wishing there were more healthy salad choices or fresh foods. That's kind of my goal here."

What should I order?

Blackened Chicken Vietnamese Taco

Fresh Off the Bun's menu reflects that objective, showcasing a selection of garden-packed banh mi sandwiches, spring rolls, pho (traditional Vietnamese noodle soup), and Vietnamese tacos and salads. From her Blackened Tofu Tacos and N'awlins Crawdaddy Shrimp Bisque, to the Vietnamese Spinach Salad with Sweet Cilantro Lime Dressing, Fresh Off the Bun dishes up one of the most whimsically delightful menus in all of Southern food truck-dom.

Count your lucky stars, folks, because Tosha's sharing one of her most popular recipes here. This caramelized pork is tender and savory, with a rich sesame favor and a tiny suggestion of sweetness. It doesn't get much better than when it's served alongside Tosha's noodle salad; but really, you can serve it with whatever dishes you usually associate with pork. It'd be hard to go wrong with this on your plate.

CARAMELIZED PORK

Makes 6 to 8 servings.

Gather it up

3 tablespoons fish sauce

3 tablespoons sugar

2 garlic cloves, minced

½ teaspoon sesame oil

1 green onion, thinly sliced

⅛ teaspoon black pepper

2 pounds pork tenderloin cut into ½-inch pieces

2 tablespoons olive oil, divided

Make it happen

Combine the fish sauce, sugar, garlic, sesame oil, onion, and black pepper in a medium bowl and whisk to combine. Add the pork pieces to the bowl and use a spoon to ensure the meat is well coated in the marinade. Allow to marinate for 15 to 20 minutes.

In a large skillet add 1 tablespoon of oil and heat on medium. When the oil is hot, add ½ of the pork. Let the pork cook until it turns brown on one side, turn, and cook on the other side until it's completely done. Repeat the process with the remaining pound of pork and tablespoon of oil. Allow the meat to rest for 5 to 10 minutes, slice into medallions, and serve.

SESAME NOODLE SALAD

Makes 4 servings.

Gather it up

5 tablespoons soy sauce

¼ cup creamy peanut butter

2 tablespoons rice vinegar

2 tablespoons light brown sugar

1 tablespoon grated ginger

½ tablespoon sesame oil

2 garlic cloves, chopped

1 (12-ounce) bag buckwheat noodles

1 cup thinly sliced cabbage

1 carrot, shredded

½ tablespoon toasted sesame seeds

2 tablespoons fried onions or fried shallots*

2 tablespoons chopped peanuts (or any other nuts if you have a peanut allergy)

Make it happen

Mix the soy sauce, peanut butter, rice vinegar, brown sugar, ginger, sesame oil, and garlic cloves in a blender until everything is fully combined.

Boil the buckwheat noodles according to package directions. Drain and rinse under cold water until cool. Shake out excess water and transfer to a bowl. Mix in the cabbage and carrot. Add the dressing, mix, and top with sesame seeds, fried shallots, and chopped peanuts.

* Available at Asian grocery stores.

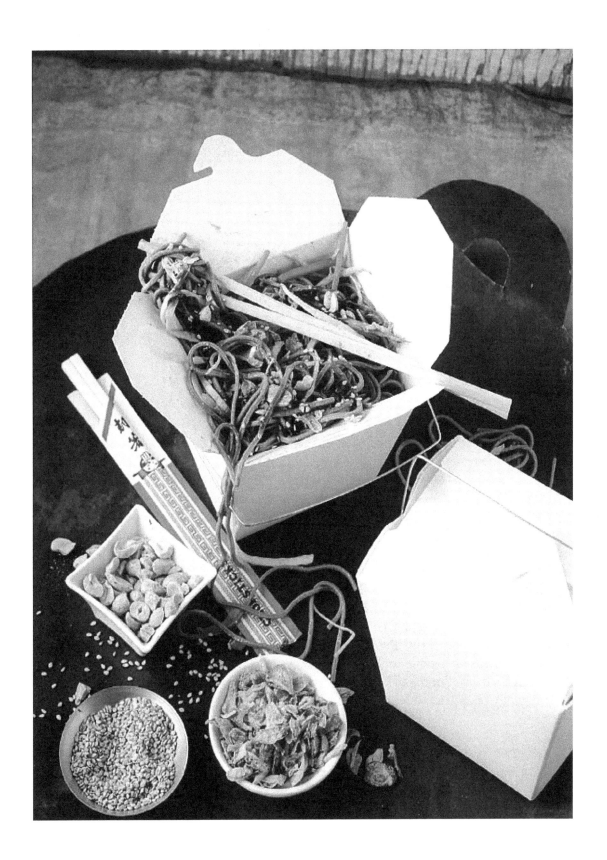

LOUISIANA

Bon Repas

Crab Cakes

BBQ Shrimp

La Cocinita

Black Bean and Roasted Butternut Squash Empanadas with Creamy Corn Sauce

Freshjunkie

Ginger Lime Shrimp Salad

BON REPAS

BATON ROUGE

Concept: Empanadas

 facebook.com/BonRepasFoodTruck

 Twitter: @BonRepasTruck

With nearly thirty years of restaurant experience under your belt, and a resume that includes some of the most upscale restaurants in the country, starting a food truck may seem like an unusual idea. Or so I thought. If my food truck road trip taught me anything, it's that career chefs love mobile dining. They're fascinated by it. They dig the idea of flexing their culinary muscles in another way by hitting the street and dishing up their creations to a new audience. Chris Wadsworth does, anyway. While he's still the general manager and executive chef at one of Baton Rouge's most upscale eateries, he also runs the Bon Repas food truck with his wife, Sommer—or, more accurately, Chris develops the recipes and Sommer runs the show out of the spectacularly pink truck that has come to be known around town for its cheekily named empanadas. There's the crawfish-stuffed Louisiana Lady, the apple pie–filled Krusader, and the famous Blue Pig, which is known and loved for its filling of Maytag blue cheese, cilantro, and Chris's handmade chorizo. For Chris, it's an effort to keep his culinary approach fresh and modern. "The food truck is an avenue for us to do something a little bit new," he said. "There are so many fresh products in the South, and everything is just really accessible here. We want to share that with as many people as we can."

What should I order?

The Blue Pig empanada, stuffed with homemade chorizo, Maytag blue cheese, and cilantro.

And in the spirit of sharing, Sommer slipped me Chris's recipes for barbecue shrimp and crab cakes. And let's be honest here—every home cook, Southern or otherwise, needs a perfect crab cake recipe in their repertoire.

CRAB CAKES

Makes 16 2-ounce crab cakes.

Gather it up

1 tablespoon fresh oregano, chopped

2 teaspoons fresh thyme

¼ cup parsley

2 red bell peppers, diced

1 teaspoon cayenne pepper

1 teaspoon black pepper

2 large onions, chopped

2 garlic cloves, minced

1 teaspoon salt

4 eggs

2 teaspoons Dijon mustard

¼ cup fresh lemon juice

1 teaspoon Tabasco sauce

1 ½ cups vegetable oil

8 cups panko bread crumbs

2 pounds back fin crab meat

1 cup vegetable oil

Make it happen

In a large skillet over medium-high heat sauté the oregano, thyme, parsley, red peppers, cayenne pepper, black pepper, onions, garlic, and salt. Allow mixture to cool. In a medium bowl whisk together the eggs, Dijon mustard, lemon juice, Tabasco, and vegetable oil. Combine this mixture with the cooled herb and spice blend, bread crumbs, and the crab meat. Mix until everything is thoroughly combined. Heat vegetable oil in a large skillet on medium-high heat. Cook the crab cakes until golden brown, flipping once, about six minutes total.

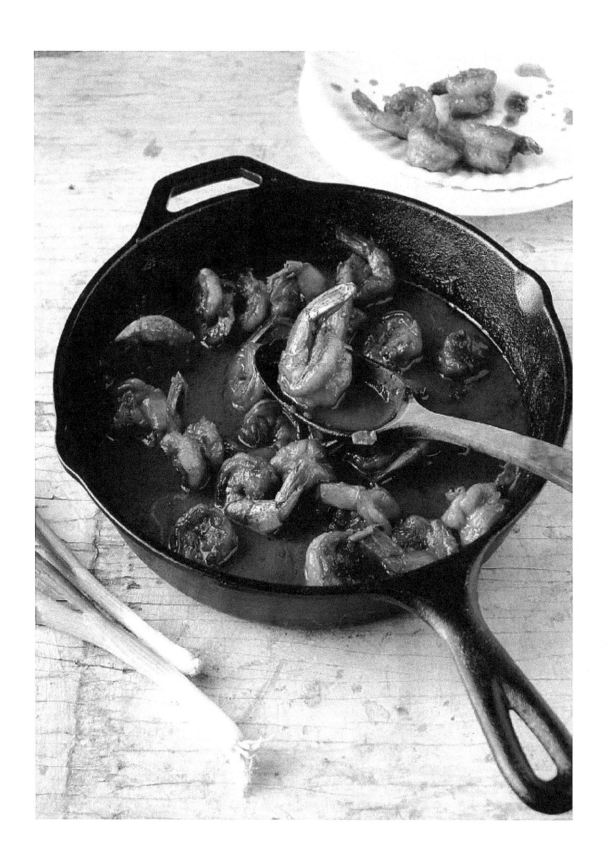

BBQ SHRIMP

Makes 3 servings.

Gather it up

25 extra-large fresh shrimp (peeled and deveined)

2 tablespoons canola oil

3 tablespoons fresh green onion tops, chopped

4 tablespoons beer

1 teaspoon chopped garlic

3 tablespoons Worcestershire sauce

1 teaspoon Tabasco sauce

1 teaspoon seasoned salt

½ teaspoon paprika

½ cup cold salted butter, cubed

Make it happen

Wash the shrimp under water and set aside. Place a large castiron skillet (frying pan or large skillet if not cast iron) on a burner and heat over medium heat. Add the oil. When the oil starts to shimmer add the shrimp. Cook until they are almost done, about 10 minutes, just before they turn pink. Add the green onion tops and cook for 1 minute. Remove the shrimp. Add the beer and reduce the volume by half, about 8 minutes.

Then add the chopped garlic, Worcestershire, Tabasco, seasoned salt, and paprika to the skillet and stir well. Cook for 1 minute and turn the heat to low. Slowly add the butter cubes to the skillet, constantly stirring to melt the butter slowly. Continue to add butter until it is all added and stir until butter is melted. Return the shrimp to the pan and coat with the sauce. Serve.

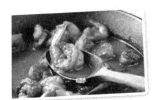

Note: This would be a great dish for a New Year's or Super Bowl party!

LA COCINITA

NEW ORLEANS

Concept: Latin American street food

⧉ facebook.com/LaCocinitaFoodTruck

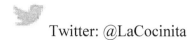 Twitter: @LaCocinita

Some food truckers develop a few great recipes, open up shop, and hope for the best. Others hit the streets, guns blazing, ready to spread the food truck gospel. Both approaches have yielded remarkable outcomes in cities throughout the South. Rachel Bellow and Benoit Angulo, a Venezuelan chef, opted for the latter method and have since become the unofficial king and queen of mobile vending in New Orleans (and by unofficial, I mean that I dubbed them king and queen). Like so many of their counterparts in this book, they caught the attention of national media outlets (the *Wall Street Journal*, anyone?), and have made as much of a name for themselves with their food truck activism as they have with their extraordinarily spiced Latin American cuisine.

What should I order?

The arepas, a white cornmeal patty, stuffed with meats, veggies, and cheeses. The braised pork variety and the butternut squash and black bean iteration are particularly memorable.

Rachel and Benoit welcomed me into their home in New Orleans's dreamy Garden District, where they fed me piping hot arepas, fresh from the fryer, and told me their story. The pair met while working at Commander's Palace, one of New Orleans's landmark restaurants. During a late-night conversation over drinks, they observed the lack of good late-night street food options in the Crescent City. Less than a year later Rachel and Benoit threw open the windows on La Cocinita, solving that problem and becoming the voice of the city's street food scene along the way. But La Cocinita, translated "little kitchen" in Spanish, is most loved for its menu. Arepas, tacos, and patacones (crispy little sandwiches made with fried plantain patties) are the perfect vehicle for any combination of meats, vegetables, cheeses, and sauces—oh, the sauces! There's guasacaca (a creamy avocado vinaigrette), cilantro and roasted green onion sauce, Latin-spiced crema, and "stupid hot" sauce, to name just a few. These original La Cocinita condiments elevate really good food to the sort of food you can't stop thinking about weeks later. Meat eaters and vegetarians alike get equal love at La Cocinita, with options ranging from braised pork and grilled steak to roasted beets and black beans.

And hey, look! Rachel sent over the recipe for a Latin specialty—empanadas, stuffed with La Cocinita's popular butternut squash and black bean filling. The *best* part? The creamy corn sauce. You'll find yourself making it to eat with more than just the empanadas. Perhaps, say, just a spoon!

BLACK BEAN AND ROASTED BUTTERNUT SQUASH EMPANADAS WITH CREAMY CORN SAUCE

Makes 8 empanadas.

Gather it up

2 cups warm water

1 teaspoon canola oil

1 teaspoon butter, melted

1 teaspoon kosher salt

1 ½ cups masa

Black Beans (recipe follows)

Roasted Butternut Squash (recipe follows)

Canola oil for frying

Creamy Corn Sauce (recipe follows)

Make it happen

To make the dough: Put the warm water in a medium bowl and stir in the oil, melted butter, and salt. Slowly stir in the masa. Knead the dough until the consistency is smooth.

To assemble the empanadas: Mix the Black Beans and Roasted Butternut Squash in a medium bowl. Roll the empanada dough into 2-inch balls. Use a saucer to flatten the balls to ¼-inch-thick circles.

Place about a tablespoon of the beans and squash in the center of the circle. Fold the circle in half, creating a pouch around the beans and squash. Pinch the center point of the outer edges together. Then use the lip of a cup to seal the edges together by pressing it downward along the rounded edge of the pouch. Peel off, then discard the leftover edges. Make sure the edges of the empanada are completely sealed, with no filling visible.

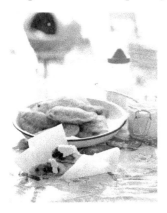

Heat canola oil to 350 degrees in a deep fryer or use about 2 inches of oil in a high-walled frying pan. Fry the empanadas, completely submerged, 4 to 5 minutes or until golden brown. Sprinkle with kosher salt and serve with Creamy Corn Sauce.

BLACK BEANS

Makes 8 servings.

Gather it up

1 cup dried black beans

4 cups water

1 carrot, diced

1 stalk celery, diced

2 garlic cloves, minced

½ onion, diced

1 teaspoon canola oil

1 bay leaf

1 tablespoon kosher salt

½ teaspoon black pepper

1 tablespoon cumin

2 tablespoons Worcestershire sauce

Make it happen

Rinse the beans and soak overnight. Drain and place the beans and 4 cups of water in a large pot. Bring to a boil and reduce to a simmer until the beans are soft, about an hour. In a separate skillet sauté the carrot, celery, garlic, and onion in the canola oil for about 5 minutes. Add the bay leaf, salt, pepper, cumin, and Worcestershire and stir for another minute. Add the sautéed vegetables to the beans and simmer for an additional 35 minutes. Remove the bay leaf before serving.

ROASTED BUTTERNUT SQUASH

Makes 2 servings.

Gather it up

1 small butternut squash

1 teaspoon canola oil

½ teaspoon kosher salt

½ teaspoon paprika

Make it happen

Preheat the oven to 375 degrees. Use a vegetable peeler to peel the squash. Spoon out the seeds and discard. Cut the squash into 1-inch cubes. Toss the squash cubes in the oil, then sprinkle with salt and paprika. Roast for 30 minutes or until fork-tender.

CREAMY CORN SAUCE

Makes 2 ½ cups.

Gather it up

4 ears of corn

2 teaspoons canola oil, divided, plus more for greasing corn

½ cup 2% milk

1 cup sour cream

2 teaspoons kosher salt

Make it happen

Preheat the oven to 350 degrees. Peel and silk the corn. Lightly grease the corn kernels with 1 teaspoon canola oil. Roast the corn for 35 minutes. Cut the corn from the cobs and allow the corn to cool. Place the cooled corn, milk, sour cream, kosher salt, and 1 teaspoon canola oil in a blender and puree until smooth.

FRESHJUNKIE

BATON ROUGE

Concept: Salads and wraps

Freshjunkie.com

facebook.com/freshjunkie

Twitter: @FreshJunkie

I met Patrick Fellows of Freshjunkie pretty late in my trip. By that point, a good three weeks in, I had gained five pounds and was sneaking up on complete meat exhaustion. Don't misunderstand—each calorie was well worth it, and I made some food memories I will treasure always. But every once in a while even the most animal-protein-loving omnivore just wants to binge on the green stuff. Patrick set up Freshjunkie to help his customers do exactly that. The menu is one big garden of goodness, served with any of Freshjunkie's imaginative scratch-made dressings—one standout being the Brickhouse variety, a Sriracha-laced potion of savory-spicy-sweet magic. Add that to a big pile of grilled asparagus and edamame, tomatoes and bell peppers, jalapeños and artichoke hearts, or snow peas and cilantro, and you've got a salad you never dreamed could taste so good. Salad isn't always necessarily the most crave-able food—even for people who happily eat a lot of it—but that Brickhouse dressing definitely ups the crave factor.

What should I order?

The Brickhouse Salad.

The idea here, Patrick said, is to "load you up on veggies with a dressing that is more flavorful than it is caloric." Nothing at Freshjunkie is especially complicated. Just good fresh salads and wraps—the concept is a straightforward respite for those customers who just want something healthy that tastes really delicious and doesn't cost a lot of money. "We ask ourselves one question," Patrick said, "'Does it make people healthier?' If the answer is no, we don't do it. End of story." After years in the restaurant industry, he realized so much of what customers ate wasn't enhancing their quality of life at all. That recognition, coupled with Patrick's own health goals as an avid triathlete, led him to develop a menu he has described as "simple. clean. fast." How many of us can say that about our lunch on any given day?

Try out Patrick's Ginger Lime Shrimp Salad and discover his secret to a lust-worthy salad. Psssst: it's all in the dressing.

GINGER LIME SHRIMP SALAD

Makes 4 servings.

Gather it up

8 cups mixed greens

½ cup shelled edamame

½ cup shredded carrots

1 bunch cilantro

1 red bell pepper, chopped

2 tablespoons sliced almonds

Ginger Lime Shrimp (recipe follows)

Vinaigrette (recipe follows)

Make it happen

Toss the mixed greens, edamame, carrots, cilantro, red pepper, and almonds in a large bowl. Refrigerate while preparing the Ginger Lime Shrimp and Vinaigrette.

Bring it all together

Toss the salad mixture with the Vinaigrette and top with the Ginger Lime Shrimp.

Patrick says: "Eat kingly!"

GINGER LIME SHRIMP

Gather it up

1 inch fresh ginger root, peeled and grated

1 garlic clove, chopped

Zest of ½ lime

1 teaspoon seasoned salt*

2 tablespoons olive oil

1 pound extra large shrimp, peeled and deveined

Make it happen

Combine the ginger root, garlic, lime zest, seasoned salt, and olive oil. Stir until well blended and toss together with the shrimp. Grill or sauté shrimp over medium heat until pink.

* Try Tony Chachere's for a Creole kick.

VINAIGRETTE

Makes ¼ cup.

Gather it up

1 lime

2 tablespoons orange juice

4 tablespoons red wine vinegar

¼ teaspoon vanilla extract (the secret ingredient!)

3 tablespoons olive oil

Kosher or sea salt to taste

Black pepper to taste

Make it happen

Zest ½ of the lime and squeeze juice from lime. Combine the lime zest and juice, orange juice, red wine vinegar, and vanilla in a small bowl. Then whisk in the olive oil. Add salt and pepper to taste.

ARKANSAS

Green Cuisine

Roasted Red Pepper and Asparagus Wrap

Quinoa Salad

The Southern Gourmasian

Chicken and Dumplings (Sort Of)

Roasted Pork and Yukon Hash

GREEN CUISINE

LITTLE ROCK

Concept: Vegetarian

rollingtomato.com

 facebook.com/GreenCuisine

 Twitter: @grncuisine

I love the menu on this little green truck, but I think what I love most about it is that it's a vegetarian food truck in Arkansas. As a Southerner, I should probably be above regional stereotypes, but I'll admit it—I've always really seen Arkansas as one of the meatiest places in the South. "The Natural State," God love it, knows its barbecue. But as I've noted before, even the most ardent flesh-eater can be tempted by the green stuff. But wait! "Green stuff" at Green Cuisine is so very different from whatever image the phrase "green stuff" conjures for you. Truck operator Lori Moore knows how to do justice to vegetarian cuisine. After quite a few years in the restaurant industry, she thought she had a general idea of what to expect. Food trucking proved her wrong . . . in a delightfully surprising way.

What should I order?

Chipotle Pineapple Black Bean Quesadilla—you'll never miss the meat!

"When I started, people told me I was crazy to do a vegetarian truck here," Lori admits. "At that point, I had been a vegetarian myself for three or four years, and I just decided that if I couldn't make it without selling meat, I'd just find something else to do."

So far, Lori hasn't needed a backup plan. Little Rock is veggie-friendly territory as it turns out. The Green Cuisine Facebook page is peppered with customers wanting to know where Lori will be next with her Philly Portobello Cheese Subs and Chipotle Pineapple Black Bean Quesadillas.

"I'm not a chef by any means, so I worked with a friend who is a good cook to come up with a menu," Lori said. "We use a few great ingredients that are well-seasoned to bring out the flavor. Most of my customers are not vegetarians, and I think that says a lot. You don't have to be a vegetarian to enjoy Green Cuisine."

She's telling the truth. The savory char on Lori's grilled veggies in this recipe give the wrap a meaty flavor. Meaty vegetarian dishes? Arkansas at its finest.

ROASTED RED PEPPER AND ASPARAGUS WRAP

Makes 4 servings.

Gather it up

24 asparagus spears

2 red bell peppers, sliced into strips

2 tablespoons olive oil

Salt and black pepper to taste

Juice of 1 lemon

4 whole wheat tortillas

½ cup hummus, store-bought or your favorite recipe

⅓ cup feta cheese, crumbled

4 tablespoons balsamic vinaigrette

Make it happen

Preheat the broiler to high.

Snap the woody ends off of the asparagus. Arrange the asparagus and red pepper strips on a baking sheet, brush with olive oil, and season with salt and pepper. Broil for about 10 minutes until the asparagus and red peppers are soft and slightly charred. Watch this process closely, being careful not to burn the vegetables. Remove from the oven and squeeze the lemon juice over the vegetables.

Bring it all together

Spread each tortilla with an equal amount of hummus. Divide the vegetables equally among tortillas. Sprinkle each with some feta and finish with a drizzle of balsamic vinaigrette. Roll into a wrap, cut into two pieces, and serve.

QUINOA SALAD

Makes 6-8 servings.

Gather it up

5 cups quinoa, cooked and cooled

¼ cup olive oil

1 cup carrots, chopped

¼ cup soy sauce or Bragg's Aminos

¾ cup parsley, chopped

½ cup lemon juice

1 cup sunflower seeds

4 cloves of garlic, chopped

2 t. honey or agave

Make it happen

Place the quinoa in a large bowl. Add the carrots, parsley, sunflower seeds, and garlic. Mix thoroughly. In a medium bowl whisk the oil, soy sauce, lemon juice, and honey. Pour over the quinoa and toss to combine.

THE SOUTHERN GOURMASIAN

LITTLE ROCK

Concept: Southern-Asian fusion

thesoutherngourmasian.com

◼ facebook.com/thesoutherngourmasian

 Twitter: @SGourmasian

If you're a Southerner, when you see chicken and dumplings on a menu you probably imagine that warm stew-y broth of shredded chicken, soft dough dumplings, and a heavy hand of fresly ground black pepper. Straightforward and no-frills. It's a dish more than worthy of its place in the comfort food canon.

What should I order?

Chicken and dumplings.

But get a load of this: the words *chicken and dumplings* mean different things to different people. Just ask Justin Patterson. After years of working in upscale restaurants in Nashville and in Little Rock's toniest country club, Justin is now exposing Little Rock-ians to a whole new interpretation of Southern comfort food: the Southern Gourmasian.

Specializing in Southern-Asian fusion, Justin serves a menu that celebrates the cuisines of the Southeast United States and the Pacific Rim in equal parts. That translates to a menu full of familiar Southern standards . . . with a spin. There's shredded pork shoulder . . . with hoisin and lime. There's coleslaw . . . accented with mango and Sriracha. There's shrimp and grits . . . with coconut and red curry shrimp. And, of course, there's the matter of the chicken and dumplings. In Justin's world, those words mean shitake mushrooms and chili sauce and a generous dusting of sesame seeds. "Every once in a while, someone will order the chicken and dumplings, and I feel like I need to warn them," Justin said. "I'll say, 'Look, this isn't Cracker Barrel. I think you're really going to like it, but just be prepared for it to be different from any chicken and dumplings you've ever had.'"

Oooh, and he's right. I sat with Justin in the one hundred-plus-degree heat of an August day in Arkansas devouring an order of the sweet, spicy, and splendidly savory chicken and dumplings in the parking lot of a bygone K-Mart. Southerners, prepare to embrace this upgrade to one of your favorite recipes, and make room in your collection for a whole new species of chicken and dumplings. Cracker Barrel will still be there tomorrow.

CHICKEN AND DUMPLINGS (SORT OF)

Makes 4 servings.

Gather it up

1 ½ tablespoons vegetable oil

4 rice cake sticks, sliced into ¾-inch segments*

1 yellow onion, thinly sliced

1 cup shitake mushrooms, thinly sliced

¾ cup cooked, shredded chicken breast

Sesame Chili Sauce (recipe follows)

1 tablespoon toasted sesame seeds, for garnish

¼ cup sliced green onions, for garnish

Make it happen

Heat the vegetable oil in a large nonstick skillet over medium-high heat until almost smoking. Add the sliced rice cakes and sauté, turning every 1 to 2 minutes until brown and crispy, 5 to 6 minutes total. Remove the rice cakes from the skillet and set aside. Add the onions to the skillet and sauté 4 to 5 minutes until browned. Add the shitakes, chicken, and the rice cakes back to the skillet and heat through, about 2 minutes. Add the Sesame Chili Sauce to the skillet and let reduce 1 to 2 minutes, stirring frequently to thoroughly coat the rice cakes. Divide among dishes and garnish with toasted sesame seeds and green onions.

* Available at Asian grocery stores.

SESAME CHILI SAUCE

Makes about ¼ cup.

Gather it up

6 tablespoons water

2 tablespoons sugar

¼ cup guilin chili sauce

1 tablespoon light-colored soy sauce

1 teaspoon rice vinegar

½ teaspoon toasted sesame oil

1 teaspoon eel sauce*

Make it happen

In small saucepan stir together the water, sugar, chili sauce, soy sauce, rice vinegar, sesame oil, and eel sauce and heat over low heat until combined and the sugar is melted. Set aside.

* Available at Asian grocery stores.

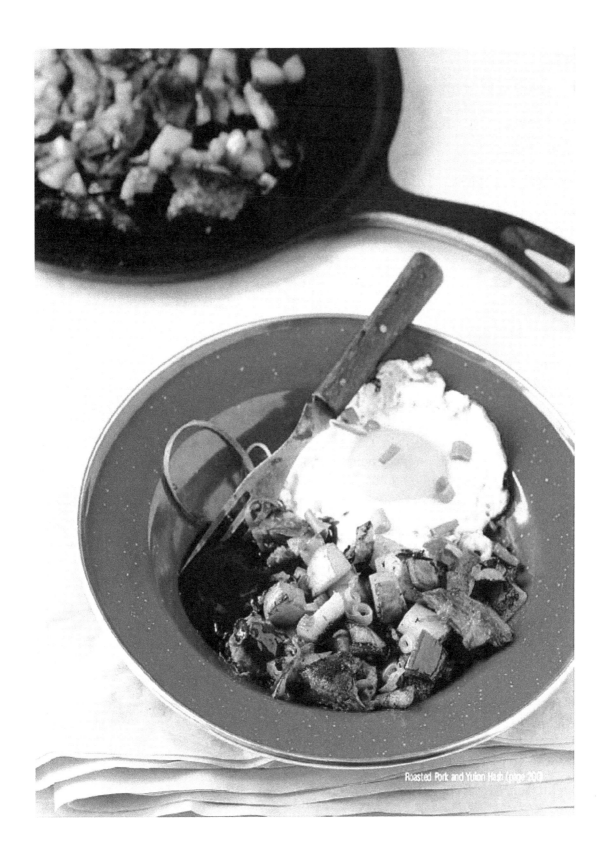

Roasted Pork and Yukon Hash (page 200)

ROASTED PORK AND YUKON HASH

Makes 6 servings.

Gather it up

1 (2-pound) pork shoulder

1 ½ tablespoons sugar

1 ½ tablespoons salt

Yukon Hash (recipe follows)

½ teaspoon sesame oil

2 tablespoons Dijon mustard

1 tablespoon molasses

4 eggs, fried to order

2 tablespoons hoisin sauce

2 scallions, thinly sliced for garnish

Make it happen

Season the pork shoulder liberally with the sugar and salt. Let rest, refrigerated, for at least 2 hours. Preheat the oven to 250 degrees. Place the pork in a roasting pan and cook uncovered for 6 to 8 hours, basting with pan juices every hour after the first 2 hours. The pork should pull apart easily with a fork. Allow to cool slightly and shred with two forks.

Bring it all together

Combine the Yukon Hash with 3 cups of the shredded pork and the sesame oil, mustard, and molasses. (You will have leftover pork.) Mix thoroughly. Portion the hash equally and sauté in a skillet over medium-high heat until lightly browned and crispy around the edges, 3 to 4 minutes.

Top each serving of hash with a fried egg, hoisin sauce, and scallions.

YUKON HASH

Makes 4 cups.

Gather it up

½ cup unsalted butter, cut into tablespoons and divided

2 large Yukon Gold potatoes, diced

1 medium yellow onion, diced

2 poblano peppers, seeded and diced

2 tablespoons minced ginger root

1 large gala apple, diced

Make it happen

Melt 4 tablespoons of butter in a skillet over medium-high heat. Add the potatoes and sauté for 5 to 7 minutes, until browned and fork-tender. Set aside. Melt the remaining 4 tablespoons of butter and add the onion, poblanos, and ginger. Sauté 3 to 4 minutes, until the onions are translucent. Add the apple and sauté an additional 3 to 4 minutes.

TENNESSEE

Jonbalaya

Jonbalaya's Jambalaya

Riffs Fine Street Food

Barbeque Jackfruit Banh Mi

Goo Goo Cluster Biscuit Pudding with White Chocolate Bourbon Sauce

Smoke et al

Fried Pickled Okra

Fiddlers Biscuits

Hoss's Loaded Burgers

The Umami Tsunami Burger

Wrapper's Delight

Triple Six Tilapia

Big Punisher

YaYo's OMG

Mahi Mahi Tacos

Gourmet Chicken Toztada

Famous Nater's

Roasted Turkey Sandwiches

Memphis Munchies

Miss Birdsong's Fried Peachy Pie

The Miss Piggie Dog

JONBALAYA

NASHVILLE

Concept: Barbecue meets Creole/Cajun

jonbalayacatering.com/

 facebook.com/pages/Jonbalaya-catering

 Twitter: @Jonbalaya

Jon Heidelberg tried a bunch of careers on for size before he landed on the one that fit just right. And if you're ever lucky enough to snag a rack of his twenty-six-hour smoked ribs, you'll be glad things worked out the way they did. This New Orleans native has been running the Jonbalaya truck, a meat-and-heat-lover's dream, in Nashville since 2010.

What should I order?

The pulled pork parfait—it tastes as amazing as it sounds.

Smoky pulled pork piled atop a bun? Sure, Jon's got that. But it's his signature pulled pork parfait that sets Jonbalaya apart from his smoker-wielding peers. Layers of pork shreds, ranch mashed potatoes, baked beans, barbecue sauce, and a bacon garnish make for the sort of portable dining that has Nashville abuzz over Heidelberg's culinary creativity. The man doesn't just smoke meat. He's constantly reimagining how it can be better.

"I'll be honest," Heidelberg said. "I want people to be blown away when they eat my food. I want it to be unlike anything they've ever tasted, and I want it to stop them in their tracks."

This is likely the sort of mind-set that produced one of his most unusual creations: Bayou Bites—a wonton wrapper filled with shrimp and grits, and flash-fried until crisp. The idea was sparked when Heidelberg spied a stack of half-price wonton wrappers at the grocery store one day.

"I said to myself, 'What's the craziest thing I can put in these?'" Heidelberg recalled of the recipe's origin.

In a nod to those Creole roots, he's sharing a modified version of his family's most beloved recipe here, as well as the namesake of his popular truck.

"Go anywhere in Louisiana and you are bound to encounter a sworn-by jambalaya recipe in every family," Heidelberg said. "Ask them to tell you what their recipe is . . . well, that's really not advised."

Family secrets aside, it's important to make enough of this dish for three days' worth of leftovers—the perfect amount of time for the flavors to achieve an ideal depth.

Use this recipe as your starting point, adjusting the ingredients to your preferences, and it could become your family's best-kept secret.

JONBALAYA'S JAMBALAYA

Makes 12 to 15 servings.

Gather it up

¼ cup canola oil

2 pounds andouille sausage, sliced into rounds*

2 white onions, diced

1 green bell pepper, diced

1 red bell pepper, diced

6 cloves garlic, minced

1 teaspoon red pepper flakes, divided

2 teaspoons celery salt

1 teaspoon Italian seasoning

Black pepper to taste

3 cups parboiled rice

¼ to 1 teaspoon cayenne pepper to taste

4 cups chicken stock

Salt to taste

1 teaspoon hot pepper sauce

2 pounds boneless, skinless chicken breasts, grilled and chopped***

Make it happen

Heat the oil in a large heavy Dutch oven over high heat. Sauté the sausage until browned. Reduce the heat to medium-high and add the onion, green and red peppers, and garlic. Season with ½ teaspoon red pepper flakes, celery salt, Italian seasoning, and pepper. Stir frequently until the onions become translucent.

Stir in the rice, cayenne pepper, salt, and ½ teaspoon red pepper flakes. Stir constantly for about 2 minutes. The rice will smell slightly "roasted." Add the chicken broth and hot sauce, reduce the heat to low, and allow to simmer until the liquid is absorbed, 20 to 30 minutes. Stir gently several times so the rice will remain fluffy. Don't over work the rice, as this will make it break down. If the liquid is absorbed, and the rice is still al dente, add water ½ cup at a time and stir gently.

Add the chicken in the last 10 minutes of cooking. Allow the jambalaya to rest for 15 minutes, gently stir, and serve.

Andouille sausage is a spicy sausage prevalent in Louisiana. If you do not have access to andouille, substitute spicy smoked sausage, or hot links.

**John says if you don't make your own chicken stock from scratch, please use some good bouillon, not just a can of stock.*

***John recommends blackening the chicken in a cast-iron skillet. On high heat, add oil immediately before adding the chicken. Season the chicken with salt, pepper, garlic powder, and cayenne pepper, cook on one side for about 3 minutes, then flip and cook on other side for 5 more minutes. If you are not comfortable with this, or want to save time, use 2 rotisserie chickens, deboned. John always recommends having your chicken broth boiling on the side. This will reduce the amount of time it takes to finish the jambalaya, which means you can start enjoying it so much faster.*

RIFFS FINE STREET FOOD

NASHVILLE

Concept: Caribbean-Asian fusion

riffstruck.com

◨ facebook.com/riffstruck

 Twitter: @riffstruck

Nashville's Great Flood of 2010. It took lives, whisked away homes, and destroyed landmarks. The flood exacted the sort of damage that makes it impossible for a place to ever completely return to the way it was, and it demanded that unique sort of goodness that always seems to emerge after a tragedy. B. J. Lofback and Carlos Davis are examples of that goodness. The two were among the volunteers helping to feed relief workers following the flood, and they realized pretty quickly that they shared a lot more in common than just a knack for goodwill. "We really hit it off immediately," B. J. told me. "I noticed that he was good with flavor in the same way I thought I was good with flavor. We ended up doing a few events together, and three years later we're still just a couple of guys doing our thing in the kitchen."

What should I order?

Go with the jerk chicken. The hype is legit.

That "thing" is one of Nashville's most popular street food menus. Riffs rolls through Nashville with an ever-changing roster of Southern standards and gourmet creations, all liberally seasoned with a broad spectrum of international flavors—particularly those from Carlos's native Barbados. On a given day, you might get the Pork Loin with Sweet Potato Kale Hash and Pear Compote. Another day you could have the pleasure of wolfing down Riffs' much-ballyhooed Jerk Chicken Nachos. Their mac and cheese gets a lot of love from the masses too.

B. J. and Carlos shared what I think is one of the most fascinating recipes in the book. Ever cooked with jackfruit? I hadn't either, but its uncanny resemblance to pulled pork in this recipe is thrilling!

And if you really want to make the ultimate "Nashville dessert," it's hard to imagine anything more Music City than Goo Goo Cluster Bread Pudding. You gotta love a dessert that's studded with big chunks of Nashville's native candy bar.

BARBEQUE JACKFRUIT BANH MI

Makes 4 servings.

Gather it up

1 cup gochujang (Korean red pepper paste)*

½ cup ssamjang (Korean seasoned soy paste)*

½ cup sugar

½ cup soy sauce

¼ cup Worcestershire sauce

1 (20-ounce) can jackfruit in brine

2 (8-inch) baguettes

2 tablespoons mayonnaise

Quick Pickled Carrots and Daikon (recipe follows)

1 bunch cilantro

1 fresh jalapeño pepper, sliced

1 small cucumber, sliced thinly

Make it happen

Combine the gochujang, ssamjang, sugar, soy sauce, and Worcestershire in a medium bowl and mix until smooth.

Pour the jackfruit into a strainer and rinse. Cut away the pieces of core. Jackfruit can produce a very convincing faux pulled pork. In a saucepan over medium heat, sauté the jackfruit pieces until hot and some moisture is lost. Do not let the jackfruit brown at this point. The goal is to replace that moisture with barbeque sauce. When pieces start to fall apart, add the barbeque sauce and simmer for 8 to 10 minutes. The sauce should reduce. Spread the jackfruit mixture over a parchment-lined cookie sheet and bake at 325 degrees for 10 minutes or so, allowing the jackfruit to dry out a bit. This is crucial to getting the pulled pork consistency.

Bring it all together

Slice the baguettes lengthwise and toast lightly open-faced in the oven. Spread each with mayonnaise and layer the barbequed jackfruit, Quick Pickled Carrots and Daikon, cilantro, jalapeño, and cucumber equally between the two baguettes. Slice each sandwich in half and serve.

* Don't let the ingredients in this recipe scare you away. Just head to your local Asian grocery store to stock up.

QUICK PICKLED CARROTS AND DAIKON

Makes 2 pints.

Gather it up

½ cup rice vinegar

¼ cup water

1 tablespoon sugar

2 teaspoons salt

½ cup matchstick-sliced carrots

½ cup matchstick-sliced daikon (or red radishes if daikon is unavailable)

Make it happen

In a small saucepan over medium-high heat, add the vinegar, water, sugar, and salt and stir until the sugar is dissolved. Remove from the heat and allow the mixture to cool completely. Pour over the carrots and daikon and refrigerate at least 4 hours. Overnight is best.

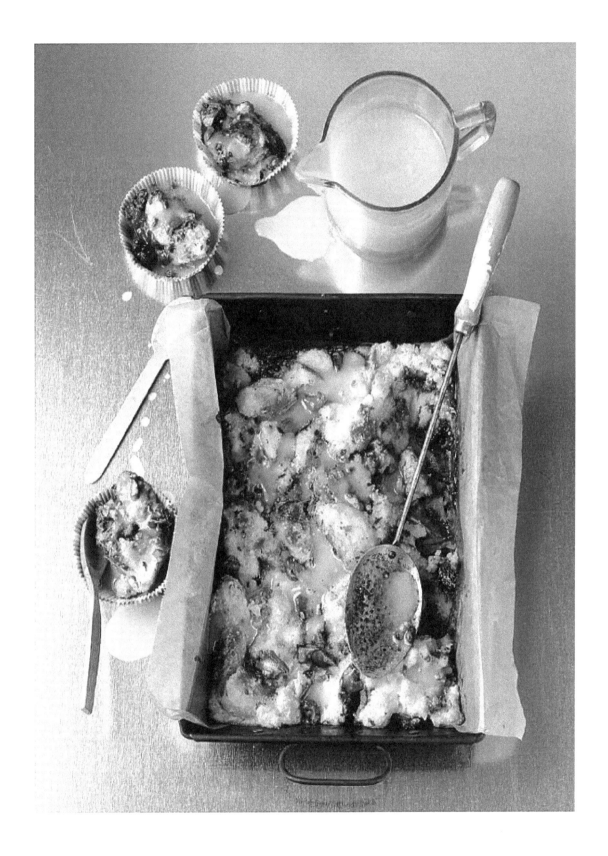

GOO GOO CLUSTER BISCUIT PUDDING WITH WHITE CHOCOLATE BOURBON
SAUCE

Makes 8 servings.

Gather it up

8 leftover biscuits (preferably homemade)

1 ½ cups buttermilk

½ cup sugar

3 eggs

2 tablespoons butter, melted

½ cup whole milk

1 teaspoon vanilla

3 or 4 (or more!) Goo Goo Cluster Supremes (the variety with pecans)

White Chocolate Bourbon Sauce (recipe follows)

Make it happen

Preheat the oven to 350 degrees. Break up the biscuits into chunks, place in a large bowl, and pour buttermilk over the biscuits. Soak the biscuits for 10 to 15 minutes, or longer if they are very dry.

In a medium bowl beat together the sugar and eggs while the biscuits are soaking. When the eggs are well-beaten and the sugar is dissolved, blend in the butter, milk, and vanilla. Pour the egg mixture over the biscuit chunks and stir until blended. Coarsely chop the Goo Goo Clusters and add to the pudding mixture.

Pour into a greased 8-inch square baking pan and bake for 20 to 30 minutes, or until it jiggles slightly when shaken. Serve warm with White Chocolate Bourbon Sauce.

WHITE CHOCOLATE BOURBON SAUCE

Makes 2 ½ cups.

Gather it up

½ cup butter

¾ cup sugar

½ cup buttermilk

2 to 10 glugs of bourbon (you'll know when to stop)

1 tablespoon corn syrup

1 (10-ounce) bag white chocolate chips

Make it happen

Place the butter, sugar, buttermilk, bourbon, corn syrup, and chocolate chips into a saucepan and bring to a boil over medium heat. Whisk until smooth. Serve with the Goo Goo Cluster Bread Pudding or on top of your favorite dessert.

SMOKE ET AL

NASHVILLE

Concept: Gourmet smoke

smokeetal.com

 facebook.com/smokeetal

 Twitter: @SmokeEtAl

Just like many of the food truckers in this book, Shane Autrey had the good sense to decide exactly what type of culinary education he wanted. That schooling turned out to be working for some of the best chefs in the country (i.e., Chef Michel Richard at D.C.'s ever so swanky Citronelle). "I saved at least $80k in culinary school tuition just by going the hands-on route in the country's best possible classrooms," Shane said. "I truly trained with culinary royalty."

What should I order?

Fiddlers Biscuits, filled with smoked chicken, Tennessee wildflower honey, and green onions.

Shane's career eventually led him to one of Nashville's landmark restaurants, The Mad Platter, where he spent three years creating a locally sourced and whimsically inventive menu. In 2011, Shane's itch to innovate led him to have an old Little Debbie truck retrofitted into what has become one of the city's barbecue destinations. *But* this isn't a pulled-pork-on-white-bun sort of barbecue truck (not that I don't love those too!). It's an heirloom-pork-transformed-into-chorizo-and-pea-meal-bacon sort of truck. But even though Shane is known around the city and beyond for his otherworldly meat-smoking skills, he doesn't want to be pigeonholed as a barbecue guy.

"We have a bountiful amount of produce and great local products in Tennessee, and it really feeds my creativity," Shane said. "The food truck is one of the last places where it's publicly acceptable to play with your food. I can't think of anything more satisfying." Shane was willing to part with the recipe for a real Smoke Et Al fan favorite. This fried pickled okra is staggeringly good. And if you can find it, using spicy pickled okra makes it even better!

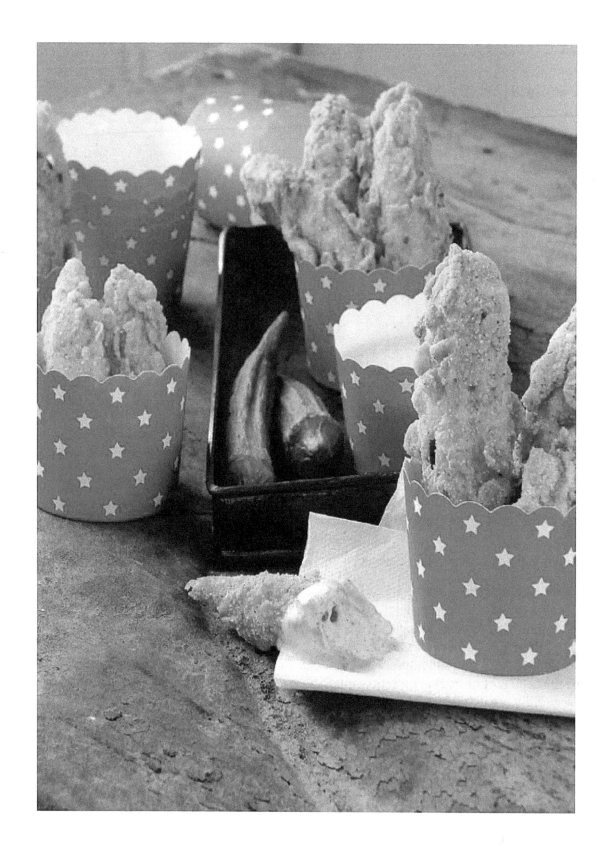

FRIED PICKLED OKRA

Makes 4 servings.

Gather it up

1 (16-ounce) jar pickled okra*

3 cups flour

3 cups cornmeal

½ cup barbecue dry rub

Salt and black pepper to taste

2 cups buttermilk

Canola oil

Bama White Sauce (recipe follows)

Make it happen

Open and drain the okra. Discard the liquid and pat the okra dry with a paper towel. In a large bowl combine the flour, cornmeal, and barbecue rub. Season with salt and pepper to taste and mix well. Pour the buttermilk into a small bowl. Dip the okra in the buttermilk and dredge it in the cornmeal mixture, shaking off excess breading.

To fry in a deep fryer: Fill a deep fryer with canola oil and preheat to 375 degrees. Carefully drop the battered okra into the fryer and cook until crispy and golden brown, about 3 minutes.

To panfry: Fill a cast-iron skillet with ½ inch canola oil and heat to 375 degrees or until the oil starts to shimmy. Fry the okra until crispy and golden brown. Be sure to roll the okra around in the skillet as it fries for even browning.

Rest fried okra on paper towels. Serve with Bama White Sauce for dipping.

* Get the spicy kind if you can find it.

BAMA WHITE SAUCE

Makes about 2 ¾ cups.

Gather it up

2 cups mayonnaise

¾ cup cider vinegar

2 tablespoons Tabasco hot sauce

1 tablespoon barbecue dry rub

Salt and black pepper to taste

Make it happen

In a medium bowl mix the mayonnaise, cider vinegar, Tabasco, barbecue rub, salt, and pepper until combined. Chill a couple of hours before serving. Use as a dipping sauce for the Fried Pickled Okra and just about anything else you like, especially chicken!

FIDDLERS BISCUITS

Makes 1 dozen.

Gather it up

4 cups all-purpose flour

2 tablespoons baking powder

1 ½ tablespoons salt

1 tablespoon black pepper

¼ cup chiffonaded* fresh sage leaves

1 cup unsalted butter

¼ cup buttermilk

½ cup sour cream

⅓ cup lemon-lime soda

Make it happen

Preheat the oven to 425 degrees.

In a large bowl combine the flour, baking powder, salt, pepper, and fresh sage. Mix together well. Using a coarse cheese grater grate the butter into the bowl. Cut the butter into the flour mixture with a fork or a dough cutter until a crumbly texture is achieved. Make a well in the center of the flour mixture and add the buttermilk, sour cream, and lemon-lime soda. Mix well using your hands until the dough just comes together. Set the dough aside in the fridge to chill and rest for about half an hour.

On a floured surface, roll the dough out to about a 1-inch thickness. Cut biscuits with a ring cutter of your desired size and place on a greased baking sheet. Bake for approximately 20 minutes or until golden brown.

* Stack the sage leaves, roll tightly, and slice across the roll, yielding long thin strips.

HOSS'S LOADED BURGERS

NASHVILLE

Concept: Stuffed burgers

hossburger.com

 facebook.com/hossburgers

Twitter: @hossburgers

Here's a life lesson for us all: good burgers are rare. Now, there are plenty of trucks, joints, and stands all over the country that use a lot of bombastic language to get you excited about what's really just an overcooked meat disc, drowned in mystery sauce and piled to the hilt with a cacophony of toppings (I'm looking at you, west coast burger purveyors!). I don't harbor any ill will against toppings. Lord knows some of the best burgers I've ever scarfed down included creamy slices of avocado. But let's all agree on one thing—the anatomy of a remarkable burger depends on a single factor: the quality of the beef. Everything else is secondary . . . no, tertiary! I'm actually unwilling to hear arguments to the contrary. Fingers in ears . . . la la la la la. That's why I really like Hoss's Loaded Burgers, where toppings are a fascinating complement and the beef is the superstar. Hoss's owner, Dallas Shaw, keeps his menu straightforward—four burger varieties on the menu at any given time, one-third pound patties of grass-fed local beef, each one stuffed with any number of cheeses.

What should I order?

The King—an homage to Elvis, topped with thick-sliced bacon, grilled bananas, peanut butter, and strawberry preserves.

There are toppings, yes—fresh veggies, herbs, and scratch-made sauces. But under it all, that beef patty is still allowed to steal the show. To my surprise, Dallas gave me the recipe for Hoss's most dazzling burger—The Umami Tsunami. If you're not altogether sure about the word *umami*, here is a (greatly) simplified explanation: *umami* is widely described as the "fifth flavor" in the salty-sweet-sour-bitter world. Umami is savory, meaty . . . making this burger aptly named. Try it out on your foodiest friends (*and* the picky eaters in your crew). Everyone will be equally impressed.

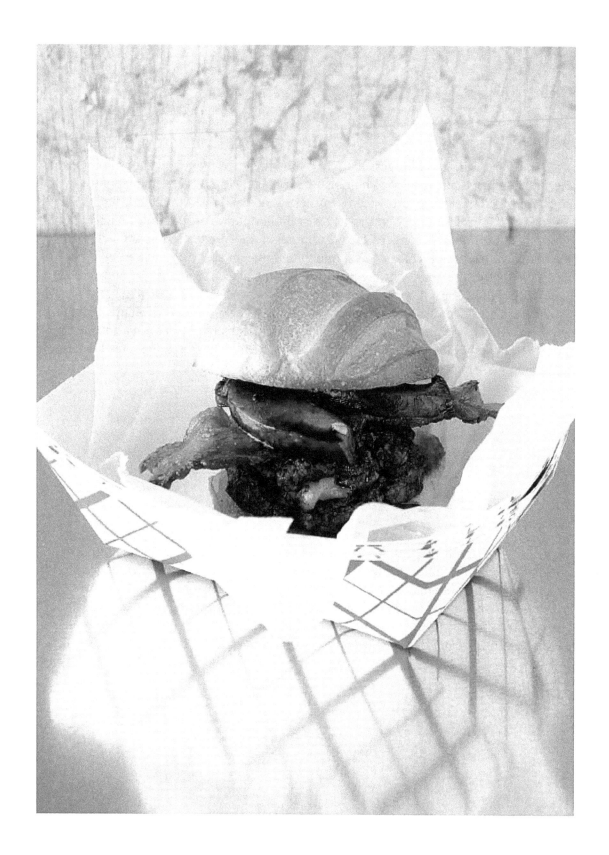

THE UMAMI TSUNAMI BURGER

Makes 3 burgers.

Gather it up

2 teaspoons sea salt

1 teaspoon black pepper

1 pound of 80/20 grass-fed ground beef (locally sourced, if possible)

3 slices smoked Gouda

3 large strips thick-sliced hickory-smoked bacon

3 (4-inch) bakery hamburger buns

Marsala Mushrooms (recipe follows)

6 tablespoons Umami Ketchup (recipe follows)

Make it happen

Either a flat griddle or a charcoal/gas grill can be used. For either method, preheat the surface to 350 to 400 degrees. While the grill is heating, add the sea salt and black pepper to the beef and gently mix them in. Try not to overwork the beef, which will result in a tough, dense burger. Using a scale, measure out 6 ⅙-pound patties and flatten them into 4 ½-inch circles. Next, fold or slice the cheese to fit in the center of 3 of the flattened patties. Press the cheese into the middle of the patties and place the other 3 flattened patties on top of the cheese. Press the 2 beef patties together, making sure to fully enclose the cheese without overcompacting the beef.

Cook the patties on the grill until cooked to your desired doneness, flipping halfway through. Hoss's Burgers are served medium to medium-well, requiring around 7 minutes of total cooking time, or an internal temperature of 150 degrees. While the burgers are cooking, cook the bacon and toast the buns. Once everything is finished cooking, place the burgers on the toasted bun bottoms and top each with a strip of bacon, 3 to 4 slices of Marsala Mushrooms, and at least 2 tablespoons of the Umami Ketchup.

Dallas says: "Be careful when you bite into the burger, as the cheese will be very hot. Enjoy!"

MARSALA MUSHROOMS

Makes 3 servings.

Gather it up

2 tablespoons bacon grease

1 portobella mushroom

1 teaspoon minced garlic

6 tablespoons Marsala cooking wine, divided (more wine can be used for a stronger Marsala flavor)

Make it happen

Heat a medium-size skillet to medium-high heat and add the bacon grease. Cut the mushroom into 10 slices and add to the skillet. Sauté for 1 to 2 minutes, stirring occasionally. Mix in the garlic and sauté for a few minutes more or until the mushrooms begin to soften. Add 4 tablespoons of the cooking wine and stir to coat all mushrooms. Reduce the heat to medium-low and allow the wine to reduce. Remove from the heat and stir in the remaining wine.

UMAMI KETCHUP*

Makes ¾ cup.

Gather it up

½ cup ketchup

1 tablespoon soy sauce

1 teaspoon white miso sauce**

1 teaspoon oyster sauce

1 teaspoon beef paste**

½ teaspoon rice vinegar

½ teaspoon shrimp paste**

½ teaspoon fish sauce

Make it happen

In a small bowl combine the ketchup, soy sauce, miso, oyster sauce, beef paste, rice vinegar, shrimp paste, and fish sauce. Stir to combine and let them sit overnight to allow the flavors to meld.

* Ingredient amounts can be tweaked for more or less of a certain taste.

** Check your local international market for these ingredients.

WRAPPER'S DELIGHT

NASHVILLE

Concept: Wraps

◼ facebook.com/pages/Wrappers-Delight

Twitter: @WrappersDLite

Nashville is good about not letting you forget that it's Music City. The moniker manages to sneak its way onto every billboard, car dealership, and bus stop bench in sight. But it's valid to note that the "Music" in "Music City" refers to plenty more than just the trademark twang and the steel guitar. In fact, Nashville has a local hip-hop scene. It may not be giving Atlanta or Los Angeles a run for the money, but there is no doubt a hip-hop subculture in the cradle of country music. Wrapper's Delight is a sort of culinary tribute to Nashville's underground hip-hop community. With a menu full of imaginatively concocted wraps, most of which are named for famous rappers, owners Sean Brashears and Gabriel Fuenmayor run one of Music City's most well-loved food trucks. Sean and Gabriel have known each other since high school, where they first discovered their shared interests in hip-hop and honing their skills in restaurant kitchens throughout the city. Between the two of them, these guys have worked in about a dozen Nashville-area eateries. So, of course, their decision to open a hip-hop-themed food truck seemed like a pretty natural move. The novelty of it, though, still really grabs me.

What should I order?

The Steakonia!

Before they opened, Sean and Gabriel sat down and brainstormed a bunch of entrees and identified the ones that easily could morph into street-food-friendly portable wraps. There's the Biggie Smalls Breakfast Sandwich, The Big L-Talian, and the Gangsta Grizzill'd Caesar.

Their best wrap? Personally, I think it's the one they shared here. The Triple Six Tilapia is one of the most unusually delicious flavor combos I've ever tasted. Fish, bacon, coconut, almond? There's nothing else like it.

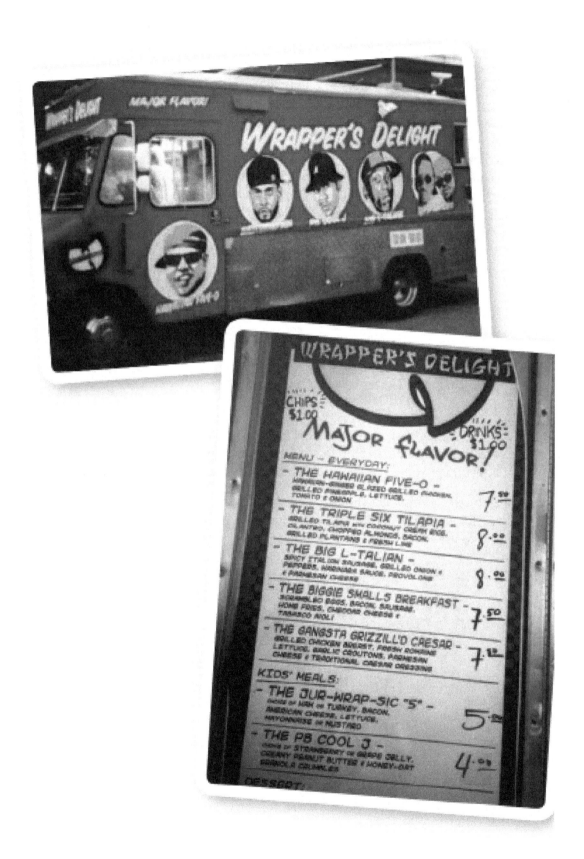

TRIPLE SIX TILAPIA

Makes 8 to 10 servings.

Gather it up

¼ cup vegetable oil

2 plantains, sliced into diagonal ½-inch-thick pieces

10 (7-ounce) boneless tilapia filets

Salt and black pepper to taste

2 limes, sliced into four wedges each, divided

10 strips bacon, fully cooked but not crisp, crumbled

Coconut Rice (recipe follows)

8 (10-inch) flour tortillas or wrappers of your choice

2 bunches cilantro, chopped

2 cups sliced almonds

Make it happen

To prepare the plantains: Place a heavy-duty skillet over medium-high heat, add the oil, and heat to 350 degrees. Add the plantain slices to the skillet in batches and fry for 4 to 6 minutes per side until golden brown. Drain on paper towels. Set aside.

To prepare the fish: Season the tilapia with salt, pepper, and a squeeze of lime. Grill or cook on medium heat in an oiled skillet on the stovetop, about 3 minutes each side. Once the fish has cooked, chop it into pieces. Mix the fish, crumbled bacon, and fried plantain pieces. Add to the Coconut Rice and mix well.

Bring it all together

Divide the mixture evenly among the tortillas or desired wrappers. Sprinkle each with cilantro and sliced almonds. Fold two sides of each tortilla inward, burrito-style, and roll. The wrap should be fully enclosed. Slice in half and serve with the rest of the lime wedges.

COCONUT RICE

Makes 8 to 10 servings.

Gather it up

1 pound medium-grain white rice

1 cup water

2 (13.5-ounce) cans coconut milk

½ cup raw sugar

Make it happen

In a medium pot over medium-high heat, bring rice, water, and coconut milk to a boil. Cover, reduce to low, and simmer for 20 minutes. Once the rice has cooked, stir in the raw sugar and mix well. Add additional sugar if sweeter rice is desired.

BIG PUNISHER

Makes 1 serving.

Gather it up

2 tablespoons honey

1 (10- or 12-inch) flour tortilla

4 tablespoons smooth peanut butter

½ banana, sliced lengthwise

Sprinkle of honey oat granola (small handful)

Sprinkle of milk chocolate chips (small handful)

Whipped cream or ice cream for serving

Make it happen

Heat the honey in a small skillet over medium heat. Spread the tortilla with peanut butter, arrange the banana on top, and sprinkle with granola and chocolate chips. Fold in half and grill in the honey until the outside of the tortilla turns golden brown. Cut in half and serve with fresh whipped cream or ice cream.

YAYO'S OMG

NASHVILLE

Concept: Tacos

yayosomg.com

facebook.com/yayosomg

 Twitter: @yayosomg

A friend asked me if I got tired of tacos during my trip. The notion of being tired of tacos amuses me. There are so many iterations of them, so many different sauces, spices, chiles, vegetables, cheeses, and protein options (what I really mean is meat . . . though I have enjoyed several really great tofu tacos). I probably downed two dozen tacos during my time on the road, and no two of them were the same. That's a testament to the versatility of tacos in general, and of the imagination of the people creating them. Chef Yayo Jimenez delivers handily in that department. The YaYo's OMG name stands for exactly what you think it does . . . as well as Original Mexican Gourmet. See what they did there? Chef Yayo's foray into food trucking began down in Miami, where he helped his brother, celebrity chef Ze Carlos Jimenez. A few years later he decided to head to Nashville, where his daughter was pursuing a music career. His timing couldn't have been better. The city's street food scene had already begun to take shape, and Nashville was nicely primed for Chef Yayo's upscale Mexican concept. My personal OMG favorite? While The Legend Taco lives up to its hype—and then some—I'm rather fond of Chef Yayo's beer-battered mahi mahi, tucked into a soft corn tortilla, along with onion, cilantro, and a splash of verde sauce. OMG, indeed.

What should I order?

The Legend Taco, with brisket, chorizo, and chicharron.

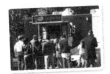

MAHI MAHI TACOS

Makes 2 servings.

Gather it up

1 (8-ounce) mahi mahi fillet, cut into even strips

¾ cup dark beer

1 cup vegetable oil, for frying

1 cup all-purpose flour

1 teaspoon paprika

1 teaspoon cayenne pepper

1 teaspoon salt

4 (4-inch) corn tortillas

Oil, for heating tortillas

Coleslaw (recipe follows)

Cilantro Sauce (recipe follows)

Make it happen

Marinate the mahi mahi strips in the beer in small bowl for 5 to 7 minutes. Heat the oil in a large skillet over medium heat until hot. In a large bowl mix together the flour, paprika, cayenne, and salt. Dredge the mahi mahi strips one at a time in the flour mixture. Gently place in the hot oil and lightly fry the fish until golden brown, 1 minute 30 seconds to 2 minutes.

Bring it all together

Heat the tortillas in a skillet with a little bit of oil. Layer two tortillas per taco. Add the Coleslaw and top with mahi mahi strips, followed by some more Coleslaw. Finish off with the Cilantro Sauce.

COLESLAW

Makes 2 servings.

Gather it up

6 tablespoons red cabbage, cut into small pieces

6 tablespoons white cabbage, cut into small pieces

6 tablespoons shredded carrots

10 tablespoons orange juice

Salt and black pepper to taste

Make it happen

In a large bowl combine the cabbages with the carrots and then mix in the orange juice. Season with salt and pepper. Refrigerate until ready to serve.

CILANTRO SAUCE

Makes 2 servings.

Gather it up

⅔ cup sour cream

6 tablespoons fresh, chopped cilantro

2 small cloves garlic

2 tablespoons fresh lemon juice

Salt and black pepper

Make it happen

Add the sour cream, cilantro, garlic, and lemon juice to a blender and puree. Season with salt and pepper.

GOURMET CHICKEN TOZTADA

Makes 4 servings.

Gather it up

Vegetable oil, for frying

8 (6-inch) corn tortillas

2 medium boneless chicken breasts

6 garlic cloves, divided

1 (16-ounce) can refried black beans

½ teaspoon salt, plus more to taste

6 medium tomatoes

1 (7-ounce) can smoked chipotle peppers in adobo sauce

1 medium onion

Black pepper to taste

½ head romaine lettuce (shredded)

1 cup Mexican crema*

1 cup shredded Chihuahua cheese**

1 tablespoon chopped fresh cilantro

Make it happen

Heat two tablespoons of oil in a nonstick skillet over medium heat. Fry the tortillas until crisp, and set aside.

Place the chicken in a pot with enough water to submerge the chicken, add 2 garlic cloves, and bring to a boil (about 5 minutes), then reduce the heat and cook for 1 to 2 minutes more. Remove the chicken from the pot and place on a plate to cool down. Don't discard the broth.

Heat the beans in a separate pan with enough water to form a soft puree. Add salt to taste.

Return the chicken broth to the heat. In the meantime, put tomatoes, 1 to 2 chipotle peppers (to increase spiciness, add more peppers), remaining 4 garlic cloves, 1 cup of water, and ½ teaspoon of salt in the blender, and mix to create sauce.

Cut the onion in half and slice each half. Add the onions and sauce to the chicken broth, and bring to a boil. In the meantime, shred the chicken and add it to the broth, reduce the heat, and cook for 2 minutes (season to taste with salt and pepper).

Spread the hot beans on 2 tortillas. Place one of the tortillas on a plate and cover with chicken, place the second tortilla on top, cover with chicken, top with lettuce, sour cream, Chihuahua cheese, and a pinch of cilantro. Repeat the above step for remaining tortillas.

* If you can't find Mexican crema, feel free to substitute sour cream or crème fraîche.

** Available in some regular grocery stores and at most international markets.

FAMOUS NATER'S

CHATTANOOGA

Concept: Southern gourmet

famousnaters.com

 facebook.com/famousnaters

Twitter: @famousnaters

When my Chattanoogan brother recommended Famous Nater's World Famous Sandwiches to me a few years ago, I was doubtful. I'm ashamed to admit it, but I just wasn't sure whether I could really take a culinary recommendation from my picky eater little brother? I had always known him as a crusts-cut-off-the-bread/no-green-stuff kind of guy. Naturally, I expected his food truck preferences to be equally timid. Turns out, my finicky little brother was spot-on. Taste buds really *can* grow up. A typical daily special at Famous Nater's might be twelve-hour braised pork with pork jus, grain mustard, parsley, and a poached egg; or maybe it's The Jimmy Carter, a pulled pork sandwich festooned with peach jalapeño relish and cream cheese. Oh, and then there's the weekend brunch selections, which almost always involve Famous Nater's *truly* famous truck-cured bacon as the focal point of *something*.

What should I order?

Absolutely anything featuring pork of any kind.

Famous Nater's namesake, Nathan Flynt, is always scheming up new ways to serve the types of sandwiches everyone already knows a little too well. For instance, a turkey sandwich with mayo is probably one of the most common lunches in America . . . except when Nathan Flynt happens to be making that turkey sandwich. Plenty of tasty turkey can be had, pre-roasted. Nathan doesn't care. He roasts his own, using a method most people reserve only for that third Thursday in

November. For his Three Little Figgies turkey sandwich, Nathan slices his slow-roasted herb-slathered turkey, piles it onto fresh sourdough, adds little pats of cream cheese, and spreads everything with his truck-made fig jam. It's an elevated version of that ubiquitous turkey-cranberry sauce sandwich at delis. Nathan's from-scratch, as-long-as-it-takes approach can be traced to the classical techniques he picked up in culinary school and in his years working with James Beard Award–winning chefs.

Oh, and when he's not slow-roasting meats and concocting jams and relishes, Nathan's sharing the recipes! It wouldn't be a terrible idea to roast up this turkey on a Sunday afternoon and treat yourself to a week of savory, herb-y lunches. Sandwiches, wraps, soups, salads. Go now and do it!

ROASTED TURKEY SANDWICHES

Makes 2 sandwiches.

Gather it up

4 slices Sourdough bread

Fig Jam (recipe follows)

1 (8-ounce) package cream cheese, chilled and sliced*

8 ounces sliced Roast Turkey (recipe follows)

¾ cup canola oil

Make it happen

Preheat oven to 350 degrees. Place one skillet in the oven. Lightly oil another skillet and heat to medium. Place four slices of sourdough in oiled skillet. Spread Fig Jam on two slices and cover other two slices with portioned cream cheese. Place sliced turkey (about 4 ounces) on cream cheese sides of bread. Flip jam side onto turkey. Take skillet out of oven and set on top of sandwiches and place back in the oven. Cook for 5 to 6 minutes or until warm and toasty throughout.

* Heat water in saucepan until it is almost at a boil. Dunk chef knife in hot water. Use hot knife to slice cream cheese. Place slices on deli paper (or wax paper is fine as well) and keep in the fridge until you're ready to make the sandwiches.

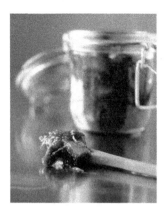

FIG JAM

Makes 1 quart.

Gather it up

2 quarts fresh figs

2 cups sugar

Make it happen

Stem and half the figs and toss in a bowl with the sugar until the figs are well-coated. Allow the figs to sit in a cool area of your house (not the fridge) for at least 8 hours (12 hours is best). Pour the fig mixture into a large pot and cook over high heat until the liquid has reduced by half. The consistency should be somewhat thick, with the figs having broken down and softened. Use an immersion blender or food processor to puree the jam to desired consistency. Cool in the fridge. Will keep for up to one month in the refrigerator.

ROAST TURKEY

Makes enough for 20 sandwiches.

Gather it up

1 5-pound fresh turkey breast*

1 bunch rosemary, or about 10 sprigs

1 bunch thyme, or about 10 sprigs

2 bunches parsley

1 tablespoon salt

1 tablespoon black pepper

vegetable oil

Make it happen

Preheat the oven to 350 degrees. Remove the turkey from packaging and pat dry with paper towels. Place the rosemary, thyme, parsley (stems and all), salt, and pepper in the bowl of a food processer and turn it on. As the herbs process, drizzle in the oil to create a slightly loose paste. Rub the herb paste all over the turkey breast and place the turkey in a tall-sided roasting pan. Cook in the preheated oven until it reaches an internal temperature of 150 degrees, about 1 ½ to 2 hours. Allow the turkey to rest for at least 30 minutes before slicing. Store leftover turkey in a resealable container in the refrigerator for up to one week.

A completely thawed frozen turkey breast will work too.

Nathan says: "We like to let ours cool all the way down to about 40 degrees before slicing."

MEMPHIS MUNCHIES

MEMPHIS

Concept: Sweet and savory indulgences

memphismunchies.yolasite.com

 facebook.com/memphismunchies

Twitter: @MemphisMunchies

Plenty of really great ideas have been born between college friends. In a sense, that's how Memphis Munchies began. In the late nineties, Tabitha Birdsong and Pamela Collins met at Mississippi Valley State University, where they discovered a shared interest: making really delicious food. Tabitha's love of sweets, Pamela's affection for all things savory, and their mutual interest in cooking fueled the dream of owning a restaurant. But, as nearly anyone can tell you, restaurant ownership is *expensive*. For Tabitha and Pamela, food trucking was the perfect entry point to their goal. So in 2009, Memphis Munchies hit the city's streets, dishing up burgers, decadent hot dog creations (Exhibit A: the recipe below), hot wings dipped in an assortment of secret-recipe sauces, and, get this—thirty different varieties of caramel apples, ranging from cheesecake and mint chocolate, to orange Creamsicle and pink lemonade. The flavor lineup reads a bit like the menu at a sno-cone stand. And as it turns out, the tart Granny Smith apple is the perfect base for pretty much any flavor you can imagine (Eggnog! Champagne! Blackberry!). Who knew?

What should I order?

The Cricket Wings, dunked in their signature Memphis Gold Rush sauce. Don't forget to pick from the dozens of caramel apple flavors either!

Tabitha and Pamela's dream was pretty simple. They just wanted to make a living selling delicious food to Memphians, Tabitha told me. Wouldn't it be great if every dream was so attainable?

Tabitha dished the secrets to two of Memphis Munchies' most in-demand treats—one savory, one sweet. Of course.

MISS BIRDSONG'S FRIED PEACHY PIE

Makes 8 servings.

Gather it up

2 tablespoons butter

4 Clingstone peaches, peeled, cored, and sliced; or 1 (15-ounce) can peaches in light syrup, drained

½ cup sugar

½ teaspoon ground nutmeg

1 teaspoon fresh lemon juice

1 (8-count) container refrigerated flaky biscuit dough

2 tablespoons water

1 (14-ounce) can sweetened condensed milk

Make it happen

Add the butter to a large sauté pan and melt over medium heat. Add the peaches, sugar, nutmeg, and lemon juice. Cook over medium heat until the peaches are soft, about 15 minutes. Remove from the heat and cool.

When the mixture has cooled, roll the biscuits out on a lightly floured surface so that each biscuit forms a 7- to 8-inch circle. Place 2 to 3 tablespoons of the filling on each biscuit circle. Brush the edges of the circle with water. Fold the circle over the filling to make a half-moon shape. Seal by pressing the edges with the tines of a fork.

Fill a deep-fryer with oil and preheat to 350 degrees. Carefully add the pies to the oil, one at a time, and fry until golden brown, turning the pies as necessary for even browning, about 5 to 8 minutes. Drain on paper towels for 2 minutes. Drizzle with sweetened condensed milk and serve immediately.

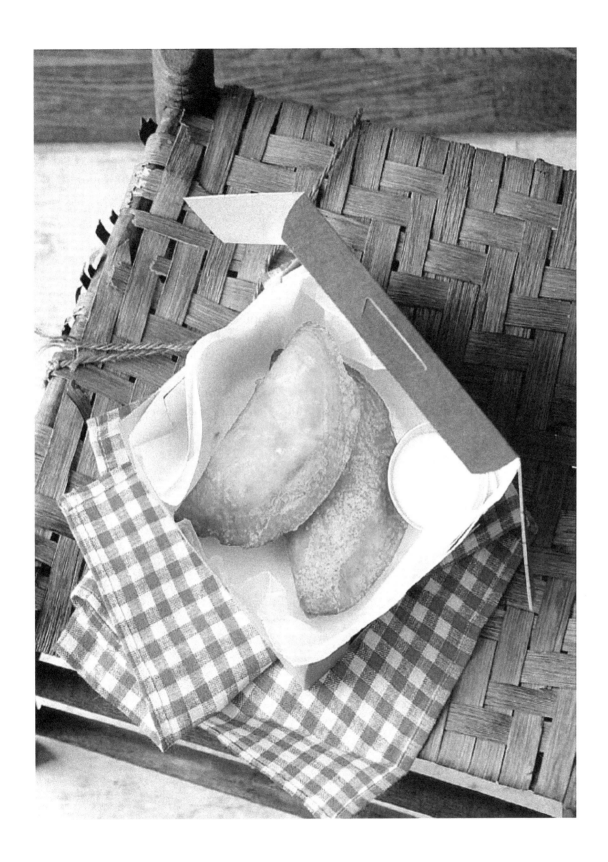

THE MISS PIGGIE DOG

Makes 8 servings.

Gather it up

8 hot dogs (regular or all-beef)

8 slices thick-cut bacon, uncooked

8 hot dog buns

1 cup pulled pork shoulder (premade in your grocer's refrigerated case or your favorite recipe)

4 tablespoons barbecue sauce

1 cup coleslaw (store-bought or your favorite recipe)

Make it happen

Wrap each hot dog in a strip of bacon and secure with a toothpick at each end. Set aside. Bring a large skillet or deep fryer with cooking oil to medium-high heat. Add the bacon-wrapped hot dogs to hot cooking oil and fry about 5 minutes until the bacon is crisp and fully cooked and the hot dogs are heated through, rotating the hot dogs several times to evenly cook the bacon. Remove from the skillet/deep fryer and set aside. Remove the toothpicks from the hot dogs and place a bacon-wrapped dog in each bun. Evenly distribute the pulled pork shoulder, a teaspoon of barbecue sauce, and a dollop of coleslaw between the hot dogs.

CPSIA information can be obtained
at www.ICGtesting.com
Printed in the USA
LVHW061123300821
696428LV00014B/361